Participatory Action Research in Health Care

Tina Koch
Debbie Kralik

With contributions from Anne van Loon
and Susan Mann

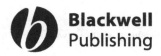

Blackwell
Publishing

Editorial offices:
Blackwell Publishing Ltd, 9600 Garsington Road, Oxford OX4 2DQ, UK
  Tel: +44 (0)1865 776868
Blackwell Publishing Inc., 350 Main Street, Malden, MA 02148-5020, USA
  Tel: +1 781 388 8250
Blackwell Publishing Asia Pty Ltd, 550 Swanston Street, Carlton, Victoria 3053,
Australia
  Tel: +61 (0)3 8359 1011

First published 2006 by Blackwell Publishing Ltd

ISBN-10: 1-4051-2416-4
ISBN-13: 978-1-4051-2416-4

Library of Congress Cataloging-in-Publication Data

Koch, Tina.
  Participatory action research in healthcare / Tina Koch, Debbie Kralik.
    p. ; cm.
  Includes bibliographical references and index.
  ISBN-13: 978-1-4051-2416-4 (pbk. : alk. paper)
  ISBN-10: 1-4051-2416-4 (pbk. : alk. paper)
  1. Action research in public health. 2. Public health–Research–Methodology.
  3. Public health–Research–Citizen participation. 4. Community health services.
  I. Kralik, Debbie. II. Title.
  [DNLM: 1. Health Services Research–methods. 2. Community Health Services.
  3. Consumer Participation. W 84.3 K76p 2006]
RA440.85.K63 2006
362.1–dc22

2005027513

A catalogue record for this title is available from the British Library

Set in 10/12.5 pt Palatino
by Graphicraft Limited, Hong Kong

For further information on Blackwell Publishing, visit our website:
www.blackwellnursing.com

Contents

Dedication

To all the people we have researched with.

Acknowledgements

We wish to thank the many people who have helped in the construction of this book. We feel greatly indebted to those whose ideas and insights preceded ours and have consequently guided our work. This book is truly a tribute to the spirit of collaboration.

We have learned alongside many people. Chapter 9 was co-authored by our colleagues Drs Anne van Loon and Susan Mann, who were the project managers for the two inquiries described. Chapter 11 was also co-authored by Dr van Loon. We extend our sincere thanks to Dr Kay Price, Kerry Telford, Pam Selim, Sue Eastwood, Shayne Kelly, Natalie Howard, Lois Dennes, Kate Visentin and Peter Jenkin for collaborating with us on the other inquiries we have described in this text. Thank you to Dr Jonathan Crichton and Penny Kearney for their careful reading and suggestions of the analysis processes. The major unnamed contributors are the people who have participated in the inquiries. Their voices are heard throughout.

Preface

This book is the culmination of a ten year research and writing partnership. It has been a joint adventure to consider ways to listen and respond to the voices of people who had previously been silent in health care. We did not conceive of this book when we started to research together, but rather have built our understandings of participatory action research in collaboration with participants. Even after many collaborative research inquiries, we continue to learn. The aim of this book is to create a story 'that is as informed and sophisticated as it can be made at a particular point in time' (Guba and Lincoln 1989:44). Knowing that this story, our perspectives and understandings will change shape as we continue to research, read, listen and learn, we emphasize that this book is a work in progress. We take this opportunity to share our experiences during the last decade and hope that you will feel stimulated to join us toward reform in health care.

About the authors

Tina Koch holds the position of Professor of Nursing (Older Person Care) at the University of Newcastle, Australia. From 1996 to early 2005, she was Director of the Royal District Nursing Service Research Unit, originally a joint chair in Community Nursing with Flinders University of South Australia.

For the past decade Debbie Kralik has researched with people learning to live with chronic illness. The research program has focused on understanding the experience of living with chronic illness and determining ways that people can learn to live well when illness intrudes upon their lives. A theory of 'transition in illness' is in the early stages of development, based on the findings of multiple inquiries. At the time of writing this book Debbie is a Post Doctoral Research Fellow on a Discovery Project funded by the Australian Research Council and jointly administered by the University of South Australia and the Royal District Nursing Service (South Australia). The title of the longitudinal research is 'Transition in Chronic Illness'.

Authorship has been rotated effortlessly and, although we have made an effort to merge our philosophies and positions, incongruence may be observed. Therefore it may be relevant to identify our individual strengths. Debbie's writing identifies most strongly with feminist theories. She leads the discussion on 'transition' and theory development in participatory action research and reflects on the role of the facilitator. Tina is guided by philosophical hermeneutics, but also continues with the debates surrounding rigour in qualitative research, further explores story telling and has developed data analysis frameworks within this text.

We are grateful to our colleagues, Dr Susan Mann and Dr Anne van Loon, whose work has enriched this book. These researchers exude attributes of care and commitment. They remind us that in the process of participatory action, so much depends on these facilitator attributes for making connections with people that have the potential to positively affect change.

1 Introduction

This book is about the use of participatory action research for inquiry and development in contemporary health practice. The aim is to position participatory action research as a vital, dynamic and relevant approach that can be engaged by practitioners and health service providers. Our intention is to emphasize that participating with people is the way to move forward towards sustainable services that evoke human flourishing. We hold strong democratic ideals, whilst at the same time recognizing that naivety cohabits with the desire for reform in health care. If naivety means we are optimistic about the potential ground swell of activity generated by participatory action as people (clients and community) come together to shape, choose and design the health services they want, we celebrate our innocence. Nevertheless, we will articulate some of the issues surrounding participatory action research in health and consider some possibilities for resolution. As with all research methodologies, approaches to participatory action research will vary with the situation and the researcher. The version of participatory action research we present is a hybrid that informs our practice as nurses researching with the community. We draw on our participatory action research experiences to present multiple contexts in our systematic studies that have used observation, the spoken word, written text and electronic communication. Our practical experience stems from our research experiences of undertaking 20 separately funded participatory action research inquiries.

Over the years we have facilitated participatory action inquiries with community members who are professionals, managers, educators and participants. These are men and women using action research to address practical questions in the improvement and development of their practice or their lives. Guided by the work of Reason (1998) we have used action research approaches to explore disruptive events in people's lives and develop ways that people can transition through the event and create a sense of continuity in their lives. Areas we have researched with people include:

- developing of participative problem solving in communities as we agree that 'the political dimension concerns people's right to have a say in decisions which affect them, and is linked with participatory economics and the development of learning communities' (Reason, 1998, p. 147);

- exploring with indigenous people their stories of living with chronic illness;
- working with people with muted and suppressed voices, such as those living with mental illness or women who were sexually abused as children;
- making contributions to nursing practice and mainstream health care.

Our aim has been to work towards greater participation in health care, so that people can contribute their ideas, and plan and partake in effective action. Our philosophy is grounded in values of democracy, equal opportunities, and education as personal development. We strive to bring issues voiced by participants into mainstream management and to government attention.

We believe that by working together with all stakeholders we can make a difference with people through participatory action research. The ability to make a difference to people's lives has been the major driving force. We view the participatory ethos as taking action towards social change and strongly believe that social justice and equity are enhanced when democratic principles guide our practice and research. Our world-view encompasses 'our total sense of who we are, what the world is and how we know it. It encompasses our sense of what is worthwhile and important . . .' (Heron & Reason, 2001, p. 4). We concur with Reason (1998), who writes that participation is a political imperative because it affirms the fundamental human right of persons to contribute to decisions that affect them:

> Human persons are centres of consciousness within the cosmos, agents with emerging capacities for self-awareness and self-direction. Human persons are also communal beings, born deeply immersed in community and evolving within community . . . we are not human without community. Participation is thus fundamental to human flourishing, and is political because, particularly in these times, it requires the exercise of intentional human agency, political action in public and private spheres, to encourage and nurture its development.
>
> (Reason, 1998, p. 147)

What has been noticeable in our experience of the participatory action research process has been the growth and development of all involved. Importantly, our research focus has not always been the identification of and dwelling on issues. Participatory action research principles direct us towards articulating strengths and the dreams and themes of 'what could be'. What is possible for the future is often envisaged through reflection and analysis of the past. We look to the past to identify strengths and possibilities because people are more comfortable journeying into the future when they carry an understanding of past events and experiences. However, with work in health care environments, nurses, medical doctors and other health care professionals are often driven by a problem-based approach to care. In our search for strengths rather than problems there exists potential conflict. It has been our experience that people who are supported, affirmed and celebrated develop the capacity to move through life's disruptions with greater ease than people who are viewed as having problems or being problematic.

Being involved in the participatory action research process has many benefits as people experience a growth and learning process. Individual and group reform has resulted in human flourishing. Participants have benefited from exposure to the participatory action research process, while researchers have also learned. Participants and researchers together have created and shared a space for working collaboratively in the development of new knowledge. Prolonged involvement with participants over time has ensured that we have listened and learned. Our world-view has enlarged and we too are enriched. Our responsibility as researchers is to share through publication of this book what we have learned.

Chapter 2 discusses the philosophical and theoretical background of participatory action research. In this chapter we describe a chronic illness research programme that has been guided by participatory principles in order to understand how people can learn to live well with illness. Chapter 3 explores the action research process of 'look, think and act' and discusses approaches to data generation. Across all data-generation processes story telling is a central activity in participatory action research.

Chapter 4 begins a comprehensive discussion about participatory action research in practice. We explore the change process using an inquiry as an illustration. This study was initiated by community nursing clinicians who wanted to respond in their practice to the needs of people who were learning to live with the human immunodeficiency virus (HIV) and the intrusion of fatigue. We describe the research process from development of the question, planning the research approach, data generation, and analysis leading to action.

Chapter 5 asks 'What happens when we learn in a participatory action process?' We illustrate and discuss the processes of group interaction by exploring data and our experiences as researchers in two inquiries. One was learning alongside older people with asthma and the other was carrying out research with people living with mental illness who also experienced incontinence. Participants with mental illness were living in boarding houses where incontinence was not tolerated; hence the collaborative development of continence promotion strategies was a challenge. We discuss the importance of context, and of people using their own knowledge and experiences in the plan for action.

We discuss how the principles of participatory action can frame community health practice in Chapter 6. This requires a shift in the problem focus towards an identification of people's strengths as practitioners work alongside them. The principles of primary health care inform this approach.

The facilitator's role and responsibilities are demonstrated in Chapter 7. We discuss the process of participatory action research and the requirement for the facilitator to be a 'resource' person and catalyst in order to assist participants to define their concerns clearly and then support them as they find their way towards action.

Chapter 8 describes some of the ethical considerations in participatory action research practice. We share the ethical concerns that emerged from two inquiries. One inquiry explored sexuality with women who live with multiple sclerosis. The other was a feminist participatory inquiry that incorporated the use of correspondence (email and letter writing) with women during a 12-month period in order to learn ways in which they incorporated chronic illness into their lives.

Primary health care principles are drivers of community development and capacity building. Two capacity building inquiries are discussed in Chapter 9, with a focus on the development of community partnerships. The first is a participatory action research project with Aboriginal Elders from rural Australia who wanted to develop strategies to bring their plight regarding the high incidence of diabetes to the attention of their community. The second example is an inquiry where we researched with women who were homeless and had been sexually violated as children. The aim was to develop capacity building strategies with these women to promote their strengths.

The aim of Chapter 10 is to stimulate debates about rigour and quality in participatory action research. We consider ways in which participatory action research work may be read as a rigorous approach. At the same time we ask whether participatory action research work is accessible, makes a difference and is sustainable. These are questions about quality. We argue that rigour and quality of participatory action research practice are co-dependent. Guidelines for reading participatory action research inquiries are offered.

There is an absence in action research literature of material for theory building. Our theoretical work on transition may be the exception. Chapter 11 discusses the process of an emerging theory of transition. Transition is a process of convoluted passage during which people redefine their sense of self and redevelop self-agency in response to disruptive life events. Whilst our participatory action research approach is primarily concerned with practical outcomes or change, theory development is a bonus, built through our exposure to the lives of the people with whom we work.

2 Philosophy Underpinning Participatory Action Research

We continue to learn and discover, reflect and make change. Like others in the study it has allowed plenty of debriefing and growth. You can do all the research in the world but without empathy, communication and excellent listening skills it just becomes another paper. You have captured insight into our lives and that came from listening, taking time to hear what we said, allowing us to talk, not belittling us, being non-judgmental, gaining trust and treating us firstly as a person and not a case number or diagnosis.

(Rhondda)

Introduction

This chapter discusses the philosophical and theoretical background to participatory action research. A participatory ethos has driven our research practice and programme. A chronic illness research programme that commenced during 1996 has focused on the experience of long term illness and understanding how people can incorporate the symptoms and consequences of illness into their lives. We have researched with both men and women who have diverse chronic conditions. A primary health care philosophy has underpinned this research programme, which has been undertaken in a community health practice setting. The key aspect of this philosophy has been researching with people; hence we have been guided by the principles of participatory action research. Participatory action research principles enable a potentially democratic process that is equitable and liberating as participants construct meaning during facilitated, group discussions. The excerpt from Rhondda that began this chapter revealed her experiences of participating in research that engaged participatory action research principles. The cyclical nature of the participatory action research process promotes reflection and reconstruction of experiences that can lead to the enhancement of people's lives, at an individual or a community level, or both.

Becoming involved in participatory action research

In an effort to understand and perhaps sequence the events that have led us to participatory action research approaches, we were reminded by van Manen (1996, p. 64) that 'the human science researcher is not just a writer, someone who writes up the research report . . . but . . . rather an author who writes from the midst of life experience where meanings resonate and reverberate with reflective being'. It is not enough to describe life meanings we hear and see, but we recognize that we are situated within our own studied worlds (Lather, 1991). We found it helpful to discuss what had led us to embrace participatory action in our lives:

Tina: What has attracted you to participatory action research?

Debbie: That's a big question! My passion for action research has been fuelled because I have experienced the process as liberating, empowering and educative. I have experienced research processes that have moved people towards reflexivity and new understandings that have brought individuals and communities into policy debate and validated their knowledge. There have been 'turning points' in my life that have led me to literally turn in another direction, toward embracing principles of participation.

Tina: My turning point was when I became conscious of the importance of listening to the stories of patients in the 1980s when I worked as a quality assurance coordinator in a large metropolitan Australian hospital. Since then, looking, thinking and acting with people has been the main motivator in both my professional and personal life. How about you?

Debbie: Well, my personal and professional life are closely entwined, so I find it difficult to talk about them as separate entities. I think I have always had a deep sense of wanting to help. My parents have told me that I had wanted to be a nurse since I was very young. I can recall feeling a little alienated in my teenage years because I did not experience the quandary of deciding what I wanted to do when I left school. Nursing seemed an entirely natural path for me even though I would be the first nurse in our family. More than twenty years later, I am still passionate about nursing. Having said this, I reflect on my earlier nursing years and clearly see my prescriptive approach to care. I was very caught up in the task orientation of nursing. I was always busy and completed more tasks than most. My patients were always spotlessly clean, shaved and nursed in an exquisitely tidy environment . . . even if they didn't want to be!

Tina: The approach to quality assurance, then and now, is largely driven by measurement of patient opinions, staff satisfaction and clinical outcomes. One measurement instrument in favour during the 1980s was the Rush Medicus Quality Monitoring Tool, which had a specific patient satisfaction component. Every day, as part of the coordinator's role, I would find myself at a patient's bedside with 10–12 randomly-structured questions from the data bank. The kinds of questions asked were: When you first came to the ward, did the nurse introduce herself? When you were first admitted to the ward, did the nurse show you how to find and use the call bell? There was an expectation that the answers to these questions would be yes, no or not applicable, dutifully recorded for further satisfaction analysis. After the patient had completed answering the battery of questions, I would linger at the bedside for a while. Discovering that patients wanted to talk about their experiences, I listened to many stories. It was evident that matters concerning patients were not those that health professionals were intent on measuring. We, as health care professionals, were not really listening to what was important to those in our care. Rather, we imposed our professional views by directing the patient's responses to conform to our quality expectations. I became convinced that working with patients was the key to caring practice and that this could be achieved through listening to their voices in the first instance.

There were similar patterns emerging in our stories. Debbie nodded her head in agreement:

Debbie: I can relate to that. I felt I was a good nurse, and indeed I knew I had a reputation of being a good nurse, an efficient nurse, but I know now that engagement with people had little place in my daily practice. I can also recall times of engaging and connecting with people in my early nursing years and I know I have made a positive difference to many people, but at that time, the tasks of nursing were the priority. They still are in many respects, but I have been enlightened by participatory ways of being with others that have impacted on my nursing practice in positive ways.

Tina: A turning point for me was my PhD inquiry (1990–1993). My study was to describe the experience of being in hospital from the patient's perspective. Emphasis was placed not only on describing the impact of the experience on patients' lives but also establishing what mattered to them about nursing. I believed that the question of what really mattered to them was the most important question to be asked. Immediately there were philosophical and interpretive questions that begged answers. How could I proceed with the inquiry? I decided each of the 14 people engaged in my inquiry would be asked: What are your experiences of being in the acute care setting and what is your story?

Debbie: So why did you turn to story telling and personal narrative?

Tina: In the early 1990s, philosophical hermeneutics was not a topic in the health literature. The interpretive questions which I pondered on for three years were about making sense of these patients' stories. When I asked a patient to tell me about his experiences whilst receiving care, I questioned how I could make sense of his story. I wondered what happened when I emphasized some aspects of his experience and ignored others. I questioned how my interests and values drove the interpretation. That others should be able to trust the accounts I offered was paramount in an era where stories were considered mere anecdote, and qualitative research was lacking in rigour. If validation with my participants had been possible, their stories may have been viewed as legitimate, but collaboratively constructing the storyline was rarely possible. Either these older people were too ill or they had died. So given that co-construction of the story was impossible, how could I re-author their stories? What would make these stories believable? I wanted to tell the story so that each account resonated with the patient's experience, but there were few guidelines to assist with creative writing. Most importantly, how could I tell these stories so that readers would understand what it was like being in hospital? And how could this new understanding enhance the health care we give? Making a difference in health care drives my inquiries. Perhaps naively, I still hold reform incentives. I know that you have similar aspirations.

Debbie: My story is a little different here, but not startlingly so. Clearly our interest in listening to people and being with people pervades. I try to carry my sense of humour on a daily basis and do try to use humour to connect and converse with others. Of course this does not mean I always use humour, even when it would work well . . . just ask our kids and my partner! My partner often says, 'If mama ain't happy . . . ain't nobody happy'. I guess that means I am not engaging and participatory 100% of the time! There have been some significant influences or turning points that have led me towards a participatory action path.

I have been influenced by feminist thought and I like to think my ways of being in the world and the ways I connect with others are framed by feminist ideology. My feminism makes sense to me. By 'my' feminism, I mean my ideas that have been shaped by my 1960s childhood experiences when authoritarian men clearly defined the roles of women within the family unit. However, I come from a family where women who are influential in my life have great substance. From a research perspective, the collaborative approach and focus of consciousness-raising in participatory action are congruent with the feminist principles that I embrace. The partnership that develops between people and me as the researcher is truly a connection through conversation. Ways of knowing are valued in participatory research as theory is generated from the experiences, lives and understandings of all participants. Participatory research is conducive to the emancipatory goals of feminism because consciousness-raising provides the way in which a greater awareness is achieved and actioned as together we engage in mutually educative and liberating encounters. Without doubt, feminism has shaped my way of being in the world.

Tina: Although we have arrived at similar philosophical positions, we want to connect with people and work alongside them towards reform at individual or community levels, the routes we have taken are quite distinct. My way of being in the world is with less humour. Given my predilection for seriousness, not surprisingly I took a move to the dour and dense intellectual environment of German philosophy. These interpretive readings were given prominence by my need to understand what happens when we listen to others. This meant at first to record my interpretive understandings, and my musings soon began to develop into a strong hermeneutical position. Among the writers who mattered, the work of Gadamer (1976, 1989) was the most appealing. I now recognize that Gadamer's influence on me was decisive. At the forefront was the ontological question of what it is to be a person. By the time I had completed my PhD study, I had delved into existential philosophy and I was beginning to answer some of the interpretive questions posed.

Debbie: How did this impact upon your thinking about being in the world?

Tina: Somewhat hesitantly at first, I saw the world as shaping me and at the same time I was shaping it. Let me explain what I think happens when interpreting. When I ask someone to tell me his story, I accept that it is his interpretation and that it comes from his own life. It comes from his background of understandings. I can make sense of his story only through comparing it with my own experiences and the experiences of others, whether real or imagined. I shape the story and I am shaped by it. A fusion occurs.

Debbie: Do you mean that it becomes a shared story . . . a co-constructed story?

Tina: Let me share an example of co-construction with Albert, an older man who was admitted to the acute care sector. The relationship between us built up over several months. I talked with him every day whilst in hospital and then visited him at his home. The story is created through the dialogue between us. I ask a question, 'What is it like being in hospital?', and I listen in order to make sense of his story. I ask further questions so that I can apprehend. When I leave his bedside,

I have a better idea of what it is like being in hospital, and I write what I have understood. I reflect on the interview process. I may choose to talk with him again, and read out to him what I have understood of his experiences. He responds. As the dialogue continues my understanding deepens. I rewrite the story and ask him again: Is this what it is like? Yes, this is what it is like. The dialogue and writing continues until we are both satisfied.

Debbie: What is to be gained from story telling?

Tina: There are changes in both researcher and participant. I am richer through understanding his story. I have initiated a meaningful relationship. I have gained insight into someone's life and I am changed as a result. I am also concerned because 'his' story is not pretty. The broad scheme of his story hovers on the emotional bankruptcy of caregivers whilst receiving care that makes him feel worthless. We agree that in his situation in a care of the elderly ward, caregivers were careless. However, being engaged in this process, I note that being heard has created in him a sense of worth and a sense of personal power. It seems that the interview process has therapeutic benefits. In the depersonalized environment of the acute care hospital someone was listening. 'I am worth listening to.' I believe the interview process stimulates reflection, and gives people a chance to think about their own situation, and working out what really matters has opened up possibilities.

Debbie: In my work, I have also emphasized that people's stories about their lives and experience should be valued, but it is important to me that the work I do contributes to action that leads to the improvement in the lives of people. A cycle of looking at and thinking about one's situation without some proactive action can be detrimental and disempowering. In my experiences, the changes people have noticed in their lives have not always happened on a large scale, but some people have acknowledged some important changes at a very personal level.

Tina: So far I can see that working collaboratively with our clients, albeit this example of collaboration is based on the dialogue between two people, opens up possibilities. The action you believe should be a consequence of looking and thinking together is not always possible. Albert was prepared to co-construct his story and in so doing he was acknowledged as a person but he did not want to complain about the service. Readmission to that setting was inevitable given his medical condition; he believed he would experience reprisals. On a personal level, being able to tell his story reversed the depersonalization he had experienced in care. There are other ways to act. One is through sharing 'his' story with those working in the depersonalized setting we described. Can the careless care he experienced, as did all the participants in my PhD inquiry, be reformed?

Tina: In the effort to reform, I share the stories of the participants inter-viewed with those who provide the health care service. Confident that these constructions would offer new understandings about patients' experiences and bring about change, I was dismayed. The realities of working in the acute setting rely heavily on routine and control of patients. When patients' stories reveal that a desire for self-liberation is an aspect of care that is important to them, service providers do not want to hear.

Debbie: Perhaps health workers hear these stories as being disruptive to their practice. Change can disrupt the continuity and certainty of the everyday. It can make us uncomfortable and open us to the scrutiny of others. To really listen to someone's story requires a preparedness to embrace something new . . . to see other possibilities. Is this where recognition of the interplay of power, both organizational and relational, comes into focus? I think this is a considerable challenge for us as action researchers.

In summary, we have noticed that the word 'participation' seems to be often used in the health literature. The merits of participatory action research can vary with both the research situation and the practitioner. At its best, the participatory action research process can be liberating, empowering and educative and can set the agenda for reform and validate the knowledge of participants. It can be a challenge to authentically embrace and practise principles of participation when working within the boundaries of hierarchical organizational struc-tures where information and decision-making are centralized (Winter, 1998). This is often the case for health services. While participation must be central to the research process, it is important that the con-struct be understood and practised as a genuine process. Participatory action research principles express participation as the central core of health practice as we move from a philosophy of doing things to clients, towards working with people to assist them to identify their own needs and formulate their own strategies to assist in meeting those needs. Habitual ways of working may need to be challenged and questioned so that innovative ways of working with people can be created. The first step is to identify what has been learned through experiences. The process of thinking about learning, the process of reflection, can be a powerful process for building self-awareness and self-confidence. Reflection increases self-knowledge and prepares people to make deliberate, well-informed choices. People engaging with the participatory action research process may find themselves on a route that takes many twists and turns; they may travel along unexpected pathways. It can take time to learn to trust the participatory action research process.

What are the beliefs underpinning participatory action research?

We now turn to the vast literature on participatory action research approaches and identify our theoretical position. As discussed earlier, the philosophy underpinning our approach reflects our concern for the ways in which we can make a difference through participatory action. Working with people to make a difference is a major theme in our work and we view the participatory ethos as facilitating action towards social change. We suggest, however, that the starting point of any inquiry is a systematic reflection on the beliefs and values driving research inquiry. Therefore our account will offer participatory action research as a methodology through describing its philosophical underpinnings and the 'world' in which it belongs.

We have chosen to introduce participatory action research by presenting issues from practice rather than 'schools of thought'; however, it is useful to understand the history and evolution of this research movement. The development of action research has been attributed to Lewin (1890–1947) as the founder of modern social psychology (Marrow, 1969). His favourite dictum was if you want to understand something then try to change it. However, in Lewin's work, participants were not involved in setting the agenda or making decisions. Stakeholders were not seen as active participants in the design of a study. For example, Lewin used action research in his efforts to change people's food habits (Friedlander, 1982).

> '. . . action research is a participatory, democratic process concerned with developing practical knowing in the pursuit of worthwhile human purposes . . . It seeks to bring together action and reflection, theory and practice, in participation with others, in the pursuit of practical solutions to issues of pressing concern to people, and more generally the flourishing of individual persons and their communities.'
>
> (Reason & Bradbury, 2001, p. 1)

Participatory action research emerged in the latter half of the twentieth century. Paolo Freire (1970), one of the world's leading educationalists, in his classic text *Pedagogy of the Oppressed* broke with the tradition of gathering data on oppressed people and instead carried out research with participants, placing capabilities in the hands of disenfranchised people so that they could transform their lives themselves. It should be noted that the methodology Paulo Freire developed was considered a threat to the established order and he was forced to leave Brazil for 20 years. In his time, however, he helped to empower countless impoverished and illiterate children. Claiming that the authoritarian teacher-pupil model failed to develop people's critical awareness he advocated an education programme based on the actual experiences of students and on continual shared investigation. Those 'learning to read and write come to an awareness of self-hood and begin to look critically at the social situation in which they find themselves' (Freire, 1970, p. 11). He argued that every person, no matter how impoverished or illiterate, can develop self-awareness, which will free them to be more than passive objects in a world in which they have no control. Often students take the initiative to transform a society that has denied them the opportunity of participation. Freire (1970) provided evidence that through working collaboratively with people this new awareness of self frees people to respond actively to change. Freire's methodology based on collaboration has had major implications for research and education in health care.

The terms collaborative inquiry and participatory action research are often used interchangeably in our work; in fact, we prefer to use the term collaborative inquiry or participative inquiry instead of participatory action research. Let us explain.

There are many forms of inquiry that are participative, experiential and action oriented (Reason & Bradbury, 2001). The action research 'family' includes a whole range of practices and approaches and the assumptions unpinning these are diverse in political, psychological and philosophical orientations. In presenting our version of practising participatory action research we draw on three orientations.

In the first version (Gustavsen, 2001), action research is the mediating discourse where the core contribution of research is 'to create relationships between actors and arenas where they can meet in democratic dialogue'. A second interpretation (Orlanda Fals Borda, 2001) explained that the tensions between theory and practice are resolved on the basis of a philosophy of life 'committed to social renovation for justice', whereas the third (Pasmore, 2001) links social and technical perspectives. Pasmore (2001) argued that new ways of thinking about research can 'challenge the dominant paradigm in research institutions, organizations and society'. We are aware that those who favour the dominant medical paradigm in health research challenge the legitimacy of participatory action. We are, however, committed to a just society and our intent is to create democratic dialogue and reform through bringing people together in a safe place. To achieve this, we are guided by social sciences and critical social theory.

Social sciences and critical social theory have provided insights from Freudian (and post-Freudian) psychology and Marxist theory. Critical theory informs a range of approaches, of which participatory action research is one, and raises critical questions about the conditions that sustain those forms of social life that are experienced as problematic by particular groups of people. The concept of hegemony (Gramsci, 1971) is important to this approach in participatory action research. The argument is similar to that of Freire cited earlier; that it is only through awareness of the ways in which people contribute to their own oppression that people can begin an empowerment process. Empowerment of people is a desirable outcome of the process of constructing and using their own knowledge.

Knowledge generation is an important aspect of the theory and practice of participatory action research. People are enabled to see the ways in which the establishment monopolizes the production and use of knowledge. This is the meaning of consciousness raising or con-scientization, a term popularized by Freire (1970). Freire's approach included learning to do by doing it. Valuing people's knowledge sharpens their capacity to conduct research about their own interests, and helps them to appropriate knowledge produced by the dominant knowledge industry for their own interests. Most importantly, it allows issues to be explored from their perspective (Reason, 1994). Hence our concern with listening to people's voices or stories is a starting point for participatory action research inquiry.

Some participatory action research approaches prioritize working with oppressed groups of people, whose issues include inaccess-ibility, colonization, marginalization, exploitation, racism, sexism and cultural disaffection (Hagey, 1997). Utilizing a participatory action research approach within this context is explicitly political when the aim is to restore to oppressed people the ability to create knowledge and practices which are in their own interests (McArdle & Reason, 2006). The intent of participatory action research is to accent the processes of collaboration and dialogue that empower, motivate, increase self-esteem and develop community solidarity (McArdle & Reason, 2006).

We have not usually aimed to adopt this larger social reform agenda as the main objective in our research. Our participatory action research group participants often include people who live on the fringes of society; our inquiries with homeless people come to mind, but we also research with people who are comfortably middle class. Although people we research with often live with chronic illness, where possible the research focus has not been specific to a medical diagnostic group but rather related to people's own construction of illness and the way it impacts upon their lives (Kralik et al., 2001b). Nevertheless, we acknowledge the work of participatory action research researchers who research exclusively with oppressed people and whose role is to actively encourage people to uncover the ways in which the establishment monopolizes the production and use of knowledge in an attempt to unveil power relations.

Feminist considerations

We have been guided and theoretically influenced by feminist and fourth-generation evaluation approaches. The primary task of feminist-driven participatory action research is to raise consciousness. It starts with a concern for power and powerlessness and aims to confront the way in which established power-holding elements of society are favoured because they have a monopoly on the definition and employment of knowledge. Participatory research is conducive to the emancipatory goals of feminist theory because consciousness-raising provides the way in which a greater awareness is achieved and results in action as the researcher and participants engage in mutually educative and liberating encounters (Kralik, 2005). Working with women as the reference group, feminist researchers tend to use a participatory action research methodology in order to achieve reform or transformational action. Key themes of feminism in relation to participatory action research are gender, multiple identities, voice, everyday experiences and power. Feminist scholars and activists are inspired by a vision of the world where women can realise their potential (Chinn, 2003). Action is the political side to feminist research; the side that says let us not simply observe and analyse these systems, but facilitate the action necessary for change to occur (Kralik, 2005).

Action research traditions were primarily associated with men. Action and feminist research problematize systematic relations of power in the social construction of knowledge. Gender is central in such power relations. This shift has pushed action researchers to grapple with gender and its meaning.

Almost every research text that discusses feminist research principles suggests that a leading goal of feminist research is empowerment of the people participating in the research through the co-construction of knowledge. There has been considerable debate among feminist researchers about the notion of empowerment and the balance of power relations within the participatory research process. The phenomenon of empowerment involves movement and change (Hutchinson et al., 1994) as 'power and knowledge are inextricably intertwined' (Gaventa & Cornwall, 2001, p. 70). Participation in knowledge development can be a way to develop awareness of issues and capacity for action (Gaventa & Cornwall, 2001). Control or lack of control between the researcher and participants can be a way of exercising power (Weedon, 1987); hence, a power relations construct has direct relevance to participatory action research.

The practice of participatory action research draws heavily on the principles and practices of feminism and other social movements (Miles, 1998). The debate in feminist literature about power relations has drawn our attention to important questions about the nature of empowerment and power relations. In her seminal book on feminist participatory research, Maguire (1987) has identified how concepts of participation and community can disguise power relations. Community and participation are concepts that can obscure patriarchal practices and class differences (Hall, 2001). We have identified five issues for discussion concerning the relations of power that have been informed by our experiences of undertaking feminist research using a participatory approach (Kralik, 2005):

- the researcher's position;
- participation and action;
- disclosure of experiences;
- consciousness raising; and
- feminist participatory research with non-feminist women.

These issues require further discussion, because how power relations are mediated is a central concept for both participatory action research and feminist participatory research.

The researcher's position

Power relations and the researcher's position within the research have received considerable attention within the literature. A debate about the researcher's position in feminist research appeared to begin with Oakley's (1981) and Finch's (1984) observations about interviewing women. Duffy (1985) proposed that in feminist research, the relationship between the researcher and the participants is non-hierarchical, reflexive and interactive, and cognisant of feelings and values. A feminist participatory research relationship targets collaboration and equality between the researcher and women participants. There exists encouragement of interactive dialogue between the researcher and participants and the mutual creation of data (Webb, 1993; Olsen, 1994; FitzGerald, 1997).

The personal experience and values of the researcher become an important component in both feminist and participatory action research. When utilizing principles from both approaches, the researcher describes and integrates his or her responses and personal feelings during the process of recounting and analysing the research participants' experiences, pain and passions. For Lawrence (1982) and Opie (1992), the adoption of a feminist viewpoint involves challenging stereotypical assumptions and maintaining a critical awareness throughout an inquiry of ways in which the researcher may influence the work. Using a feminist research approach has created the space for us as researchers to join our own experiences as women with those of the women who have researched with us (Kralik, 2002, 2005). In this way we locate our own voice during the research process, and learning, personal reflection and knowledge growth become integral to the research process.

As researchers who represent a privileged, white middle-class, we have been challenged, disrupted (Opie, 1992) and sometimes silenced (Bhavnani, 1988) when we have researched with women from diverse culture and backgrounds. We have been challenged as our ways of seeing and being in the world have been expanded and we have been disrupted as we have come to understand the worlds of women, which have sometimes been at odds with our own. We have been embraced by their insight and wisdom, developed from living a life disrupted by illness, extreme violation (abuse) or social stigma.

Ribbens (1989) argued that an empowering research approach is intended to allow the voices of those involved in the inquiry to speak more clearly. To achieve this, Ribbens (1989, p. 590) suggests researchers need to acknowledge their position within the research process:

> 'Ultimately we have to take responsibility for the decisions we make, rather than trying to deny the power that we do have as researchers.'

We suggest that this may be achieved if the researcher, together with participants, develops strategies that enable the inquiry to be used as a platform for voices to be heard. One participant shared her experiences of reading a research paper for publication:

> 'I have just skimmed through the first few pages (of the findings) and I am so choked up. I am very moved to have our story told and that the day is getting closer for others to hear our cry for understanding and compassion but certainly not pity or sympathy.'

Women who we have researched with, over time have come to develop a commitment and an ownership of the direction of the inquiry. Often we notice a change in their language as they refer to 'our research'. When asked the question, 'What has surprised you about participating in a participatory action research inquiry?', Heather responded:

> 'The cohesion in our group, at least with what I think of as the core group – those of us who chat almost daily. The friendship and camaraderie, the understanding and support have been incredible. The care for each other's needs has been truly wonderful. Being part of a *community* . . . where the members live the best lives possible with the limitations they have. In our community we share each other's joys and suffer with each other's sorrows and difficulties. It is also a community where the members understand each other's trials and disappointments. It has been a life-enhancing experience.'

Maddie also participated in a recent participatory action research inquiry and shared her experiences of involvement:

'It has been very freeing in a way. I have learnt through our group that it is okay that I have a chronic illness, that it's okay that I need to have a sleep through the day. It has also been confrontational at times to really look inside myself and face facts. I wouldn't have missed this opportunity for anything.'

Participation and action

Participation has been central to the progress of our inquiries as together we have created the storied accounts of people's lives. It is proposed that feminist participatory research embraces the notion of intersubjectivity, with the researcher and participants mutually creating data (Olsen, 1994). There is debate about the extent to which participants are involved in feminist participatory inquiry and the nature of their involvement. It has been our experiences, particularly when researching with women who are learning to live with long term illness, that participation is often influenced by the capacity of the individual and that validation often occurs when participation is acknowledged and celebrated rather than expected. Participation often encourages a close relationship between action and research (Lather, 1988; Cancian, 1992). Creating the space for participation is discussed in later chapters.

Lather (1988) writes of the use of an action-research approach to encourage students taking a women's studies course to engage with the emancipatory perspective she saw as the aim of the course. Mies (1983) wrote of a feminist participatory action research project that included street demonstrations with the purpose of awakening local consciousness to the need for a woman's refuge. This project has been described (Lather, 1988; Speedy, 1991) as an example of women becoming empowered to take action through a research project:

'The purpose was to empower the oppressed to come to understand and change their own oppressive realities.'

(Lather, 1988, p. 572)

Throughout our inquiries, people have participated in different ways and with different degrees of intensity and commitment. For some, involvement has been erratic because the time available to devote to the inquiry was impacted upon by other events happening in their lives or exacerbation of illness. For others, a personal commitment to the purpose of this inquiry was apparent. This commitment has often increased as people have identified therapeutic benefits gained through involvement in PAR research. The consequences of their involvement fit comfortably with the feminist principle that participants should gain benefit from their research involvement. A researcher's judgement and expectations about the degree of participation may create an imbalance of power. Acknowledgement and celebration of participation, however, creates the space for greater engagement in the inquiry processes.

Disclosure of experiences

Many participants have described how the telling of one's story, and the feeling that someone is listening, can be an empowering and therapeutic experience. Men and women have expressed that they had lived with corrosive silence because they perceived that people had not wanted to hear their stories, stories that have been so intense and personal for them. This silence had resulted in some people postponing any personal analysis of their experiences. Through the course of a participatory inquiry, when stories are finally told, people often find new meaning in their experiences. Mishler (1986, p. 119) suggested that there are ways that researchers can communicate with participants that both empower and encourage them to speak in their own voice:

'When the balance of power is shifted, respondents are likely to tell stories . . . interviewing practices that empower respondents also produce narrative accounts . . . Through their narratives people may be moved beyond the text to see the possibilities of action. That is, to be empowered is not only to speak in one's own voice and to tell one's own story, but to apply the understanding arrived at to action in accord with one's own interests.'

Through the process of creating the space to give voice to the voiceless, some people have felt validated and empowered and experienced an increased self-awareness that has often been the impetus for change. For Kerry, involvement in the research process seemed to have a therapeutic benefit:

'Working with you has been so beneficial for me personally. I was thinking back to a time prior to my involvement in our project . . . and all that has happened since then in terms of my understandings and perceptions . . . and I know I will be eternally grateful to you and to the other women for my growth.'

Some participants have responded with intensity to their experiences and made known their strong desire to have their voices heard. This strong desire contributed to their disclosure of rich descriptions of their experiences. People have described how they were pleased they had the opportunity to share their experiences for the purpose of research so that others who live with illness, and health professionals, may gain a greater understanding of the experience of illness. For some participants their experiences with illness had left them with a decreased self-esteem and a sense of inadequacy. For these people in particular, the telling of their story through a participatory action research inquiry provided them with a sense of purpose, which was experienced as empowering. They were satisfied that their story would be useful and that therefore their experiences were validated and had a purpose. Rona explained:

> 'I have appreciated the feedback I have been given, at no time have I felt any criticism or patronizing; this was very important to me. So many times I have encountered well-meaning people, particularly in the medical profession who dismissed what I felt was important to me.'

There have been several instances in our inquiries when people have disclosed highly personal information. Denise said: 'I was thinking how amazing it is that people pour out their innermost, private and personal details to a stranger. I told you things I've told no-one!' Seibold et al. (1994) had identified this as a dilemma in feminist research and expressed concern over the balance of power relations when women revealed intimate details to the researcher, and then had no control over analysis or how the researcher used their stories. It has been important for many participants to have the opportunity to read the way that they are portrayed in the final report and in future publications. We have also co-authored publications with participants.

Consciousness raising

Feminist research aims to raise the consciousness of people in general and of the participants specifically (Stanley & Wise, 1983). Consciousness raising is enabling people to view the world in a different way and is based on knowledge gained. Henderson (1995, p. 63) offered a description of consciousness-raising in feminist participatory groups that has relevance to our participatory action research experiences when she said:

> '. . . in feminist groups, women experience a shared sense of reality and a shared sense of oppression; they become conscious of their problems as group problems rather than as their own individual problems.'

Feminist and participatory action researchers try to use consciousness-raising about the context of people's experience as a tool for narrowing the distance between researchers and participants by generating reciprocity and collaboration (Lather, 1988; Olsen, 1994).

Reciprocity lessens the hierarchical nature of the researcher's position within the research. We have used several approaches, such as sharing our own experiences, assuring participants of their right to refuse to answer any questions, and sharing the constructions of other participants rather than imposing our own meanings on the experiences of others. Reciprocity affects all participants and gives individuals, including researchers, a sense of their identity (Banister, 1999). It is educative to consider the lives we have lived and the moments of particular significance within our lives, which play a part in shaping our ways of being in the world (Parker, 1998). Participants have become aware of their position or situation through the research process and they then aim to change their situation. People explain their social reality in personal accounts of their lives, and the themes emerge from their shared experiences (Holloway, 1997). The changes in the health situations of people, particularly in relationships with health professionals, become evident as participants position themselves as central and in control of their health and illness care. Beverley explained that having to understand her responses to illness meant that she placed her experiences with illness into the context of her life and this has had wide-ranging benefits:

'This anonymity has created a certain sense of safety and has aided in my honesty and openness. Following writing about an area I had previously kept to myself, I have found that I am then able to discuss the issue with those close to me. So not only have I gained more insight into how I really feel about having a chronic illness and life impacts this has had, but those who support me are also benefiting as they can understand me better and therefore more effectively provide the support that I need.'

Participatory feminist research with non-feminist women

Throughout the process of our inquiries we have been aware that our notions of power might not be helpful to participants. Furthermore, without the voice and direction from participants themselves, our notion of power as researchers may be misconstrued as empowerment to do as we want, not empowerment for participants to express their own views, or take their own actions. Bowes (1996) concurs that there is a danger that researchers might misappropriate their view of empowerment by leading participants in a certain direction in order that they may analyse their situation in terms of gender and power relations. We have experienced that in some situations, participants may actually be disempowered and further disorganized in the short term by the participatory action research process. This situation might occur if researchers undermine a woman's immediate coping strategies, which do not involve any long-term structural change. Angela, a participant, said:

'I don't know who I am. I have never known who I am, because it's always been about them. I've moved into violent relationships because it was about them and that meant I didn't have to face me, because I don't even know where I begin and end, let alone who I am. My whole life I have worn masks and made myself what I felt other people wanted me to be. Now I don't have a clue who the real me is, or even if there is a real me.'

After a life of extreme violation at the hands of others, Angela was beginning to explore her identity and sense of self through participatory action research group processes. We suggest strongly that participants themselves have to be free to draw their own conclusions about their position in their lives. To impose feminist ideology on a participant may impose on their reality and forge changes for which they are not prepared. Mary-Ann, who participated in an inquiry, wrote about experiencing a particularly difficult time:

'I was told how bad I was for not being with my children. I did not need to be told that because I felt bad enough for letting them down . . . I have now asked everyone to pretend like I am dead.'

When participants engaged in the participatory action research process choose an action to take in their lives, it is often decided upon after much guided reflection, validation and affirmation from group processes. The participatory action research process guides participants to explore the experiences that bind their past and future together to give them a sense of continuity. This exploration reveals to them the current ways they cope with change and how these may have been militating against their capacity to choose how they define themselves (a person with illness, a person who is worthy). The complexities and challenges in people's lives must be taken into account when considering the issue of the balance of power within participatory action research and feminist research.

Fourth-generation evaluation approaches

Fourth-generation evaluation (Guba & Lincoln, 1989), in an effort to address managerial dominance within organizations, applies a constructivist methodology to evaluation where all stakeholders have a voice (ideally). The starting point is the lived experience of people, and the idea that through the actual experience of something, people come to understand it as reality. Thus in fourth-generation evaluation the knowledge and experience of people is directly honoured and valued. Fourth-generation evaluation unites the evaluator and the stakeholders in an interaction that creates the product of evaluation. Indeed, evaluation is a process that involves evaluators and stakeholders in a hermeneutic dialectic relationship. Similar to participatory action research in intent, fourth-generation evaluation is a methodology for an alternative system of knowledge production based on the people's role in setting agendas, participating in data gathering and analysis, and controlling the use of the evaluation outcomes. Guba and Lincoln (1989) also comprehensively described the differences between positivists and constructivist paradigms of research, and provided practical steps and processes in conducting fourth-generation evaluation.

Nevertheless, we have identified five characteristics that distinguish participatory action research from other research methods (Cancian & Armstead, 1990; Cancian, 1992; Reinharz, 1992; Henderson, 1995; Seng, 1998).

(1)   Participatory research involves participation by the people involved in the research at all stages of the research process. The issue being researched originates with the individual or the community. Participants may be involved in developing the research design, generation of data and analysis, and then participate in the dissemination of the research findings. The nature of participatory research suggests that there exists a partnership between the researcher and research participants.

(2)   Ways of knowing are valued in participatory research as theory is generated from the experiences, lives and understandings of all participants. Theorizing helps individuals explain their lives by exposing false ideologies. The act of theorizing may create opportunities for change in the lives of those individuals participating and can lead to a wider scale social transformation in collective lives.

(3)   There is a focus on empowerment and power relations in participatory research. People's awareness of their own capabilities and capacity is strengthened by their participation in the research process. Empowerment is incorporated into the process of the research by identifying the potential for the imbalance of power in the research relationship and seeking to take action to address this inequity. By acknowledging the power imbalance in the researcher/participant relationship, the process can be empowering for those involved and allows the imbalance to be investigated as a part of the research process (Henderson, 1995).

(4)   Participatory research views consciousness-raising as the core of this approach. The research process may be educative for both the researcher and the participants because together they generate data. All people involved are researchers and committed learners.

(5) The aim of participatory research is to create social change, which addresses the inequality of power distribution. It aims to affect the lives of those who participate in the research (including the researcher) in ways that the participants see as being beneficial to their lives. The goal is to improve the lives of those participating in the research. The social change begins with the participants (including the researcher) and may often end there as well. It is recognized that change may be limited to consciousness-raising or behaviour changes in the individuals who participated in the research.

Participatory action research often appeals to clinicians and others working in practice environments because it translates quickly into action so that change can be observed during the process of research. It is a flexible, albeit systematic, methodology that is ideal in the constantly changing clinical environment. A participatory action research approach is often perceived by practitioners as having immediate relevance because variables are acknowledged and considered rather than controlled. The individual and/or community is seen in context and collaboratively all those involved in the research construct the meaning of and implications for the issue under research and devise possible solutions. The individual or community is perceived to be a partner in research and all people involved in the inquiry seek common ground in defining the issue, determining the direction of the research and moving towards action.

A selection of approaches

In recent years, the creative capacity of researchers worldwide has resulted in the development of a selection of participatory reflection and action approaches. Many approaches have existed in other contexts, and have been borrowed and adapted for the inquiry being undertaken. Others are innovations arising out of situations where researchers have applied a diversity of approaches, the context and the people themselves giving rise to development of a novel approach. This was certainly the case for our use of correspondence when researching with people with chronic illness. The expectation of people who have chronic pain to attend a prearranged group meeting was unrealistic. We needed to devise a research approach where people could participate when able, and with minimal intrusion into their lives. Participatory action research approaches in a health setting could involve the following.

Direct observation. Go and see and experience for yourself. This is often effective for understanding the context of a situation. Immerse yourself in the situation. A critical awareness of personal biases is needed, however, that may have resulted from our past education, culture and experiences.

Seek out the stakeholders. This may seem obvious, but can be an aspect not considered. Who are the key stakeholders of this research? Seek understanding of their experiences/contextual knowledge and issues and invite their participation. Discover their needs and priorities.

Story telling. Ask questions of people that promote story telling. What have been their experiences in the past? What do they feel has worked? What hasn't worked? Why?

Case stories. Examples may be the story of an individual, a family or a community.

Group meetings. These can be with a community, or a specific group of people that have common features, concerns or issues. Group conversations may be a source of rich data generation and can provide the impetus and motivation for action.

Understanding context through presence. For example, being with participants in the area that they live. This enables a feel for context, observing, asking, listening, discussing, learning issues, seeking issues, solutions, opportunities, and mapping and/or diagramming resources and findings.

Timelines and change analysis. Listing major events and experiences with approximate dates; people's accounts of the past, of how customs, practices and things close to them have changed.

Shared presentations and analysis. Where local people and/or outsiders, especially at community meetings, present maps, models, diagrams and findings.

Contrast comparisons. Ask one group to analyse the responses from group two and vice versa. This could be useful in situations where gender awareness is important.

We have used all of these approaches, and often have incorporated several approaches within an inquiry. Participatory action research is about inclusiveness in the construction of knowledge that leads to action. What these approaches have in common is a participative world-view. Each of these approaches encourages us to examine our intent and behaviour and the taken-for-granted assumptions, structures and relations that shape the way we live and work (Maguire, 1996). Issues include the need to examine the philosophical underpinnings of the research approach taken, the legitimacy of participatory action research in a medically and managerial dominant world and the way in which story telling and our representation of voice can be trusted. Emphasis on rigour and quality is paramount if the participatory action research process is to be accepted by its critics as a legitimate research inquiry. In Chapter 10 we dwell on the notion of rigour and quality of action research inquiries.

3 Participatory Action: What It Is

A change in our lives because of an illness causes us to think with our soul and heart instead of with our other means of learning. We are confronted with the need to change dramatically because nothing fits with our reality anymore.

(Kerry)

Participatory action research is a process in which 'we', researchers and participants, systematically work together in cycles to explore concerns, claims or issues that impact upon or disrupt people's lives. Collaboratively we reflect on ways to change situations or build capacity. We act according to self-devised plans to bring about social reform on a macro level or continuity into individual lives on a micro level. The systematic approach to data generation and analysis, its cycles of validation as we collaboratively decide what counts as data, and its clear auditable documentation, make participatory action a research approach. The cyclical nature of the participatory action research process promotes reflection and reconstruction of experiences and stories that can lead to the enhancement of our lives, at an individual level, community level, or both. Together we decide on the shape of the outcome, which may be a resource, a research report, a web site, a book for public readership, published papers or ideas for further research.

There are numerous definitions of participatory action research (Street, 1995; Reason, 1994; Wadsworth, 1998; Stringer, 1999; Reason & Bradbury, 2001; Gergen, 2003; Green et al., 2003). Our definition has evolved during the last decade and is based on our practical experiences of researching with more than 300 people who live with chronic illness. Stringer's (1996 and 1999) participatory action research has guided our thinking and research approach because it is community orientated and as nurse researchers working in the community, it made sense to us and the other participants in the research.

According to Stringer, a fundamental premise of community-based action research is that it commences with an interest in the issues of a group, a community, or an organization. Its purpose is to assist people in extending their understanding of their situation and thus resolving issues that confront them. Community-based action research is always enacted through an explicit set of social values. In modern, democratic social contexts, it is seen as a process of inquiry that has the following characteristics:

- It is *democratic*, enabling the participation of all people.
- It is *equitable*, acknowledging people's equality of worth.
- It is *liberating*, providing freedom from oppressive, debilitating conditions.
- It is *life enhancing*, enabling the expression of people's full human potential.

Look, think and act

The action research process works through three basic phases (Stringer, 1999):

Look – building a picture and gathering information. When evaluating we define and describe the issue to be investigated and the context in which it is set. We also describe what all the participants (educators, group members, managers etc.) have been doing.

Think – interpreting and explaining. When evaluating we analyse and interpret the situation. We reflect on what participants have been doing. We look at areas of success and any deficiencies, issues.

Act – resolving issues. In evaluation we judge the worth, effectiveness, appropriateness, and outcomes of those activities. We act to formulate solutions to issues.

We were attracted to participatory action research because its process has been shown to be equitable, transformative and liberating for participants (Stringer, 1999; Stringer & Genat, 2004). The PAR approach favours consensual and participatory procedures that enable people to set the agenda for discussion by prioritizing issues that are important for them, to reflect on their experiences, and to devise actions that they perceive as being both possible and meaningful within the context of their lives. We use a variety of data generation strategies when researching with people, including one to one interviews, group work, telephone conversations and email conversations. Each of these strategies will be discussed in more detail in the following section.

'Look, think and act' describes a systematic, cyclical action process. The look process starts with creating the space for the person (or group) to have a voice, tell a story or describe a situation. Creating the space for voice involves ensuring a comfortable environment, safety (establish group norms), authentic listening, allowing people time to talk and responsiveness without judgement. There is a strong possibility that narrating one's experience can help people make sense of their lives (Sclater, 1998; Kralik, 2000). This means that researchers need to be cognisant of developing ways to enhance listening, seeing and writing. People live stories, and in their telling of them, reaffirm them, modify them, and create new ones. Constructions of experience are dynamic and new understandings emerge as we begin to make sense of our complex social world.

Looking means the group (or individual) observing the setting or the situation, gathering information, and defining and describing the issue. The framework of the issue or situation is established. People will offer different perspectives, reflecting who they are, their culture and their life experiences. From a researcher's perspective, looking may also mean building a picture of the research setting and relevant events, identifying the key stakeholders in the research, and locating relevant documents, literature and records.

Thinking is stimulated as the facilitator asks participants to reflect on the emerging picture, contributing their own story and those of others to ask: 'What is happening here? Why are things as they are?' The facilitator encourages participants to engage in discussion and dialogue, so as to develop mutually acceptable accounts describing their experiences. In this way participants can learn from the experiences of others, yet at the same time, each person has an opportunity to be heard. Facilitators and participants collaboratively attempt to create meanings through conversation. Together we compare and contrast our various interpretations. Stories and analysis occur concurrently, which enables identification of emerging understanding from early data to guide the subsequent group discussions. Feedback to participants is ongoing. In terms of rigour, critical to validation of the data-generation process (or the story line), the main constructions from the previous group session are presented and confirmed at each gathering or conversation. In short, thinking refers to exploring, analysing, interpreting and explaining events, story lines and interpretations.

When contemplating action, participants question what is important in their lives and consider the options that are available to them. Story analysis occurs during successive individual interviews or when the groups are in progress. Constructs, issues, concerns and strengths are extracted, shared and discussed. Co-construction of stories and validation with participants is ongoing throughout the inquiry. When working with multiple groups of people focused on the same topic, it is important to retain both the distinctive features of each group and also to find recurring constructs across groups. Involvement of participants ensures constructs are congruent with their life experiences and as such, enhances the rigour of the inquiry. The simplicity and order of the look, think and act process motivates people and clarity about an issue emerges. Often firm friendships develop between participants and the group process is sustained after the researchers have left the inquiry. Heather said:

'The friendship and the support have been important. I now have several good friends that I did not have two years ago. These friends are extra special as I know when they ask how I am that they really mean it. To have non-family members who can celebrate my small victories and commiserate on the bad days is a big help. The encouragement I have received from these friends is beyond price. I am so glad our group will continue.'

The participatory action research process translates knowledge into action. Central to this process is a cycle of critical reflection and learning. Reflection is about learning to understand our human situation and ourselves as we try to construe meaning out of the experiences and situations of which we are a part. Chinn & Kramer (1999, p. 171) used the term 'personal knowing', which is 'an unfolding process that is grounded in the context of everyday experience, in relationship with others'.

Theoretically in the participatory action research cycle, there is a conceptual difference between the 'look, think and act' elements. In practice, however, these conceptual differences begin to dissolve and merge. Instead what happens is that people engage in many cycles of reflection on action, learning about action, considering possibilities and then devising new informed action which is in turn the subject of further reflection (Wadsworth, 1998). During conversations, people absorb new ways of seeing or thinking in the light of their experience, leading to new actions. With practice, these become the focus of discussion, further reflection and group self-understanding. Change from action often does not happen at 'the end' of a participatory action research inquiry, but rather it happens throughout (Wadsworth, 1998). During the participatory action research process it often occurs that the focus of what needs to change will shift over time as people alter their understanding of what is really important to them. Denise revealed the shifts in learning she experienced when involved in the participatory action research process:

'I learned a great deal of facts and information from the research and experiences of others. I had some of my own ideas and knowledge re-affirmed by others with the same experiences or who could understand completely. I learned that we are not alone in our trials and tribulations, yet we still have to contend with others who have not experienced a chronic illness and more, those who have not experienced any illness. I learned to question, and to have a high regard for the ideas of resilience and adaptability.'

We will draw on our experiences and learning while undertaking research inquiries in the community. Inquiries have taken place in a variety of settings and although the 'look, think and act' process guides our research, we have identified a number of data generating approaches. Working principles of participatory action research guiding these inquiries include relationships, communication and inclusive participation (Stringer & Genat, 2004). These principles are based on the assumption that people are self-determining authors of their own action, who can and do learn to reflect on their world and their experiences within it. Everyone involved in the research inquiries has contributed to collaborative thinking, decision making and idea generating, underpinned by notions of reciprocity and respect for each person and their self-agency.

One to one interviews

Interviews are particularly useful for gaining in-depth understandings about the personal context behind a participant's experiences. They also give both the researcher and the participant the opportunity to pursue in-depth information around a topic or issue. There have been several research studies in which participants have requested one to one interviews with us in addition to participating in the participatory action research group processes. Some people may be reluctant to speak out in a group situation, unable to attend a group due to pain, fatigue or immobility, or perhaps want to share with a researcher an intimate aspect of their story.

Participant stories are generated through successive, one to one in-depth interviews. Relationship building is fundamental to the interview process. The researcher engages with the participant in a way that promotes comfort, trust and safety. The time and place for the interview should be comfortable for the participant. Consider alternative places to a clinic, such as the person's home, a café, restaurant or community centre. Research is a sociable process (Stringer & Genat, 2004) so it is important that researchers identify themselves, discuss the area of interest and the background to the research, and follow ethical guidelines with regard to informed consent. Participants must be assured that they can stop the interview at any time or choose not to answer a particular question. This is very important when undertaking interviews around sensitive topics.

During the first interview the person is asked to tell a story and some prompts or direct questions are asked. These questions are usually general, broadly based on the topic under focus and conversational in tone. For example, 'Tell me about your illness . . . I don't know much about it.' During subsequent interviews, questions are shaped by three participatory action research components (look, think and act) and usually become more focused on the issues the participant has raised: 'Tell me more about . . .'. The key processes here are observing, listening, questioning, feeding back and combining challenge with support within the context of conversational dialogue.

Not all questions are asked during the same interview, as each conversation builds upon the previous, actualizing the look, think and act process. One can only tell a few parts of a story at a time; hence feedback is provided before another interview is commenced. When engaged with story telling, reality is created in the moment and there are multiple realities. Sometimes the same story is told with an emphasis on different aspects of experiences, or the telling of the story shifts as new understandings emerge. With informed consent, interviews are audio recorded, transcribed verbatim and analysed. In addition, the researcher's field notes or journal provide further interview data.

Telephone conversations have followed a similar data generation and analysis process. Participants have stated that telephone interviewing was convenient, not intimidating, not time consuming, and overcame the difficulty with mobility that some people experienced. Important to the participatory action research process is prolonged engagement, so that meanings can be articulated and underlying features of people's experiences unpacked. Telephone interviews do not in the main represent an action research process; however, it is one approach that can be combined with other methods of research engagement. Telephone interviews can be one way of staying in contact with participants between meetings, to inquire after participants' well-being and to promote connection during a longer research process.

During the interview, people are invited to share their experiences, their accounts, their events and their stories throughout the participatory action research process. Looking, thinking and acting invite active reconstruction of the story line. When we listen, it is noted that the PAR process encourages people to focus on aspects of their lives that were previously taken for granted.

Look, think and act cycles are appealing because they have meaning for people in their everyday lives. The appeal of this process seems to be its simplicity. Prior to being involved in participatory action research processes, some participants were already using a similar process to work through confronting issues. People for whom the 'look, think, act' process was new, worked towards adopting it as a way to develop the capacity to take action in their lives. In this way, the participatory action research approach can be a systematic learning process in which people act deliberately through being responsive to possibilities and opportunities. It is a process of using critical reflection to inform action, and working with people so that action becomes praxis.

Story telling

Across all data generation processes story telling is a central activity in participatory action research. The analysis requires us to follow a story's movement at an individual level and at a group level. At an individual level, we think about the self as a valued social construction that is reproduced time and time again in everyday life. This image of the self has evolved over time. The self is not only something we are but involves an active constructing of an ongoing, ever changing story. It has been observed that the ability to tell and be heard has served as a basis for people to make sense of their relationships and of their responses to illness. We have observed that a shift in a person's self-identity is evident. Why transition is significant and the way in which movement from disruption to continuity can be detected has been the focus of analysis. It has been our primary research focus to explore the way in which people reconstruct continuity following an unexpected disruption in their lives.

It is possible to follow the language people use to talk about themselves and their experiences and show that shifts in identity occur over time. However, while identities such as age, gender or race may be 'fixed', other identities reflecting personal qualities are a matter of construction during interaction. Self-identity is a dynamic process that evolves from an ongoing interaction between the individual and the social environment. Others involved in constructing identity, such as labelling or stereotyping, may do so in ways over which the individual being identified has only limited control. Turning to our research findings with people learning to live with chronic illness, having less control over the way others view the individual may be related to living with a chronic illness when changes in bodily appearance become apparent. In fact, several researchers have conceptualized chronic illness as precipitating identity shifts (Bury 1982, 1991; Charmaz, 1983; Yoshida, 1994). The position taken by the authors is that the self and identity are co-constituted. We cannot ignore the post-modern conceptualization that we embody multiple identities that shift and change as we influence and are influenced by our circumstances, learning and social contexts (Holstein & Gubrium, 2000).

Often when people are engaged in the participatory action research process they reflect on what they have learned through relationships with other people in their lives. People learn that they interact with many people who play an influential role. These people could challenge, criticize, motivate, inspire, understand and accept, or judge them. Certainly for some people, reflecting on past experiences has been an uncomfortable process. The researcher may need to be ready to refer participants to appropriate counselling services or other supports, such as tribal elders, healing circles, support groups or psychologists. Through this activity, participants inevitably begin to gain a deeper understanding of themselves, their supports and their abilities. Often, by reflecting upon difficult or unhappy relationships or events, people might even be able to see these interactions in a new way. People may be able to look beyond the challenges confronting them to see new opportunities and possibilities in their lives. When we research with people we reflexively explore personal and social change and/or transition. Dynamic stories of the self are created. Our intention is to capture that movement. Rhondda wrote of her participation in one inquiry:

> 'It has been a learning and discovery time, time to reflect, time to make changes and like others in the study it has allowed plenty of debriefing and growth.'

Participatory action research groups

There are many theories surrounding group work. During the 1960s there was a popular theory that groups have discernible, linear development stages (Tuckman, 1965). Our experiences, however, are that each group is different and group processes are not necessarily linear. This may be because most groups start as a collection of individuals bought together with little to connect them other than the common focus of the research inquiry. The participants in many groups 'click' spontaneously with the right mix of personalities, skills, resources and motivation. For other groups, time, energy and thoughtful research initiatives are required to develop connections. Of course, communication is the core activity that enables a group to develop and proceed with its intent. Communication can only flourish in a safe environment where group members can share their thoughts, and receive support and encouragement when they risk being honest. People will rarely take risks in a group situation where they do not feel safe. Why would we expect them to? Controlling or judgemental behaviour from other group participants will reduce trust levels.

When we convene a participatory action research group, we carefully consider the location of where the meeting will be held. We consider issues such as access (stairs, ramps), car parking, public transport routes, seating and room layout. Often, we provide transport if this is considered necessary to enable participants to attend. Accessibility is important, as is the time of the meeting. For example, when researching with parents of young children, it may not be wise to plan group meetings at the time of day that school finishes.

It is important that the group develop norms that permit participants to share and work through uncomfortable emotions and experiences. During the first meeting we discuss the development of group 'norms'. We ask all participants to consider what is important to them in a group environment. The group norms are devised from their responses and often revisited at subsequent group meetings. Creating a safe environment in which we can share intimate information is paramount and needs to be talked about at the outset. As a group, we talk about not embarrassing someone by laughing or making light of an experience that they are sharing. Discussion centres on the importance of respecting each other's opinions and experiences. Confidentiality of identities within the group is always stressed, that is, whatever is said within the group stays within the group.

We have usually invited 10 to 12 participants to share their experiences about an issue or topic of their choice. We have learned that between 10 and 12 participants promotes cohesion between people, allows the time and space for people to have a voice, and is workable in terms of recording conversations and events occurring in the group. Meetings have been usually held weekly or fortnightly, and up to 10 meetings are held with each group, lasting between 2 and 3 hours. Availability of research funding and pre-determined time-lines has often placed a constraint on the number of meetings and the duration of the research.

The time of the meetings and the setting are mutually agreed upon. We have learned the importance of ensuring there is time before the group meeting commences and after the meeting finishes for participants to chat and get to know each other. This encourages the relationship building that is so important within the participatory action research process. Often we provide food and refreshments because the offering and sharing of food also creates a relaxed, friendly atmosphere. Having refreshments on the table can reduce the formality of a 'round table' layout.

At the first meeting with participants we get to know each other as we each introduce ourselves and share some information about our background and why we joined the research. During the first meeting, participants are often dependent or tentative and looking for guidance about what will be acceptable to the group. The issue of inclusion or exclusion becomes important and the facilitator is required to keep a watchful eye on the developing group dynamics. People are invited to place issues on an agenda for discussion but in the first instance they want some direction. We may ask questions to stimulate thinking, such as: What is important to you? What would you like to discuss within the group? What do you hope to achieve from participating in the group?

During the course of subsequent meetings participants are invited to share their story. They tend to place emphasis on aspects and experiences that are important to them. Personal agendas begin to be revealed and cohesion within the group becomes evident.

As the participants share their stories the group begins to form an identity. When all participants have been heard, and this could take several sessions, questions around 'look, think and act' may be prompted as we begin to reflect on what has been shared. Participants begin to assist each other to explore common strengths, problems and issues, and to formulate experiential accounts of their situations. Participants therefore are co-researchers, and they collaboratively decide on actions, either as individuals or as a group. At the subsequent participatory action research meetings the findings from concurrent analysis are fed back to participants for reflection, discussion and validation, and further discussion ensues. In this way, findings are shaped collaboratively. The group processes can promote a sense of validation of experiences. Space is created for talking about issues that are otherwise silenced. Common threads of experience emerge. When researching with women about the changes they had experienced in their sexuality since having multiple sclerosis, Vera said that she felt she had a voice for the first time and it had been comforting for her to hear the experiences of others:

> 'I didn't know if others have a problem or only me . . . I know that I am not alone. I was not asking [others about sex] because it was private, but I have learnt that I am looking, thinking and acting too.'

Story telling and analysis are both systematic and collaborative. Conversations are audio recorded with consent. In addition, a person with excellent typing skills processes the participatory action research group conversations verbatim. This means that we have immediate access to data for concurrent analysis. Often a researcher will write some notes during the conversations, capturing context or inaudible events in the group. Ideas are extracted and discussed by the research team before the next participatory action research meeting. Analysis of the data follows pre-established protocols that are discussed later.

Email correspondence

While involved in the participatory action research process we have utilized email correspondence and a listserv. Currently, we are researching with two groups, one of men and the other women (2003–2006) who are learning to live with chronic illness. Our aim has been to understand the experience of living with chronic illness and to further theorize how people can live well while illness has a place in their lives. Participants have diverse and sometimes complex symptoms that they are learning to live with. The medical diagnosis has not been a categorizing characteristic for participants in this inquiry but rather we have relied upon the participants' own construction of illness and the way it has impacted upon their lives (Kralik et al., 2001b). The research will attempt to answer the question 'What is transition?' Whilst transition or 'moving on' is identified as a life process, here we are concerned with researching with people over an extended period of time to understand the way chronic illness impacts on the lives of people and the way in which they respond.

During this research we intended to have prolonged engagement with participants. Data generation has spanned 2 years and analysis has occurred concurrently with group discussions. In this way, participants have been central to the analysis processes.

When groups were first convened, participants were asked to provide a biographical account in response to some broad questions: What would you like the group to know about you? Tell us about an incident or episode that really changed your life. How do you feel about changes to your body? How has illness affected the way you live, socialize, play, study or work? What are the important issues for you?

The group conversational processes have developed over time into a 'learning circle', which has fed into the cycle of 'look, think and act'. Learning circles are usually virtual communities that are an effective and practical method of learning and social change (Hiebert, 1996). The main distinctions between a learning circle and a discussion group are that learning circles are usually more focused, based on common resources and have action outcomes.

Participants learn at their own pace, reflecting on their own experiences and understandings, without a researcher or an expert leading the discussions. A researcher facilitates the group conversations by asking questions, prompting reflection and sometimes providing alternative ways of thinking. When the group progresses, the need for active facilitation becomes less, as participants themselves begin to take up these roles. Exchanging ideas and experiences enhances learning because it is inherently a social process of constructing shared understandings. Denise shared her experiences of participating in a learning circle:

'My experience has been one of learning about how others live with a chronic illness and I found out lots of information from their research and experiences of living with a chronic illness. This then helped me to realize I was not the only one having to contend with uncertainty, the actual impact of the symptoms of the illness and unpredictability. My experience included improving in empathizing with others, a less cavalier approach to thinking when others were ill or disabled that "Oh that would never happen to me". I have been influenced by group members to search for information, have a more assertive approach with doctors and paramedical people and to never give in to living life as a victim.'

The facilitated groups provide structure and process to the learning circle and create a shared way of understanding. The process of reflective correspondence held meaning for Rhondda, as it helped put events in her life into perspective and create a vision for the future:

'It has meant a great deal to me in being able to truthfully write about all that I have been through and the aftermath. In a way it has given me a better understanding of who I am and where I am heading. I have got rid of some heavy baggage I was carrying around. Areas that had been put to rest but never resolved have had an airing. I can see by reading back that I am a worthy person, I have a fairly clear insight into where I get my strength from, how I have overcome tragedy and how I coped with a life threatening illness . . . It has been a long learning journey, one I wouldn't have missed for anything.'

The 'action' from people has not always been obvious (i.e. in the sense of social reform), due to constraints such as pain and mobility; however, making sense of experiences has been a priority (making sense is often the act). Clearly, when we make sense of our experiences through the reflection processes of looking and thinking, possibilities for action become ignited. Developing these online communities with people has been about creating a shared way of thinking about our worlds.

Collaboration

Collaboration is a word that is often used and from our perspective means working together for a greater purpose. It means finding common ground with others for whom the research is important (research participants, key stakeholders, clinicians, community members) in order to work towards a common vision. Collaboration, however, does not always mean harmony or always being in agreement with others, but it does mean creating a relationship where shared interests are advanced through the processes of dialogue and cooperation. When collaborating, neither person's perspective dominates but rather a shared perspective emerges through dialogue; hence, collaborative relationships are inherently creative.

People who collaborate trust one another, and trust requires time; hence our assertion that participatory action research generally requires prolonged engagement with participants. It is less likely that strangers will collaborate than people who have worked together for a longer period of time.

Regardless of the data generation approach used, whether it has been one to one interviews, groups meetings, or email list serv discussion, we begin with story telling and refer to this phase as 'looking'. Asking for biographical accounts or simply 'story telling' has engaged researchers' attention as a method of accessing the personal world of illness (Gergen, 1991; Frank, 1993; Koch et al., 1999; Kralik, 2000; Holstein & Gubrium, 2000). Whilst we refer to our transition research, particularly researching with people who live with chronic illness, we regard transition as a life process and have found story telling to be meaningful in every participatory action research process regardless of focus or approach.

Research participants initiate and determine the salient questions; hence, they co-create the findings. Assertiveness and listening are complementary aspects of facilitating collaboration. Both are essential elements for creating the space in a group for collaboration and communication. Listening and asserting, however, are not the same as hearing and speaking. When we listen to others, we are allowing their points of view to predominate in our awareness, but when we assert, our point of view prevails. To collaborate, we must balance the two perspectives and allow the synergy from the competing views to emerge as insight. Sometimes this is the 'ah-ha' experience that comes with newfound awareness or understanding of a situation.

Participatory action research is collaborative because those people responsible for action are often directly involved in improving the situation or circumstance that brought them to the inquiry. During the participatory action research process, the collaborating group is often widened from those most directly involved, to engage as many as possible of those affected by the practices concerned. Most importantly, the people who are affected determine what constitutes findings and decide what forms the findings will take. Finally, they determine the representations and the shape of the research outcomes. As it is a participatory research programme with people, theory is developed collaboratively.

Theory building

There is an absence in the action research literature of material for theory building (Dick, 2004). Our work on transition may be an exception. The cyclical nature of the participatory action research process promotes reflection and reconstruction of experiences and stories that can lead to the enhancement of people's lives, either at an individual level, community level, or both. As discussed earlier, our involvement in participatory action research inquiries with people who live with a chronic illness has enabled us to build theory from participatory action research. Building theory collaboratively with community dwelling participants has been a distinguishing feature of our research programme.

The aim is to make a difference in health care; hence, we believe that theory is defined by its practical effects. In each of the inquiries we question common assumptions held about the experience of living with chronic illness. In so doing we have discovered that theory is often a confrontational critique of common sense notions and a challenge to biomedical constructions of illness. Theorizing means attempting to show that what we take for granted has been historically constructed. Whilst it is a critique of common sense it is also an exploration of alternative constructions. In order to make a difference, we need to show what our theory disputes. The theory must offer ways in which people, research participants, significant others and health care professionals, can think differently about living with chronic illness. The effect we desire through theorizing is to shift people's views. Guided by participants, reshaping our practice to listen, learn and understand is the core of the reform we envisage.

4 The Participatory Action Research Process in Practice

Participatory action research involves people reflecting on and theorizing about their practices. As a starting point, this requires people to be inquisitive about understanding the relationships and forces between circumstances, actions and consequences in their lives. Participatory action research is suited to identifying issues in clinical practice and working collaboratively with others to develop potential solutions in order to improve practice (Meyer, 2000). Participatory action research principles foster the gathering of clinicians' and clients' intuitive knowledge and experiences; hence, because findings are generated with participants, the findings resonate in people's lives. The metaphor of voice is common to both feminist and action research (Macquire, 2001). A voice with which to share one's experiences with others, to learn with others, and a voice for practitioners and community members when they collaborate in the production of knowledge (Winter, 1998).

Change processes can occur slowly; hence, the impact of engaging with a participatory action research process can resonate long after a researcher has left the field. We have found that it is important that the outcomes of participatory action research are not judged in terms of the magnitude of the change achieved or the action undertaken, because participatory action research often makes its impact as a process of ongoing learning and awakening. Judy shared her experiences of story-telling during the participatory action research process, providing a new perspective:

'It has been interesting for me to tell my story because I now realize just how far I have come in accepting my illness and that I can enjoy life in spite of it. I now feel that regardless of my physical life, I will still have an exciting future.'

In the following section we illustrate this using a research practice example.

A Participatory action research inquiry with people living with human immunodeficiency virus and fatigue

The aim of this study was to go beyond objective clinical assessment and explore the experience of fatigue and self-care strategies with adults who live with human immunodeficiency virus (HIV). This research inquiry was initiated by clinicians who wanted to respond to the needs of people with HIV who were learning to live with the intrusion of fatigue in their daily lives. District nurses who held the position of clinical nurse consultants (CNCs) drew attention to the issue of fatigue experienced by people living with HIV. It was suggested that fatigue was one of the most prevalent, yet under-reported, under-recognized and under-treated aspects of living with HIV. Fatigue has been described as tiredness that is unrelieved by a full night of sleep (Lee et al., 1994; Ancoli-Israel et al., 2001). Adults who had been diagnosed with HIV for at least 12 months and who perceived that fatigue was a issue in their lives were invited to participate in the research (Jenkin & Koch, 2004).

HIV is being increasingly recognized as a chronic illness because of therapies that may lengthen the lifespan of people infected by the virus. These therapies have benefits but can also have side-effects. The changing clinical and social focus of HIV as a chronic illness has implications for the way that nurses work alongside people with HIV, hence the impetus for this inquiry. Previous research had revealed fatigue to be a prevalent, yet under-reported, symptom of the chronic illness experience (Kralik et al., 2003), but research exploring the experience of HIV-associated fatigue has not been extensively reported and as a consequence may not be well understood.

Together with participants, we explored self-care strategies and identified the catalysts and constraints to self-management of their condition. Analysis was concurrent to data generation so as to ensure a feedback loop to all people involved in the inquiry. This feedback loop with participants of emerging understandings enhances the rigour of analysis, and also creates the opportunity to build our (participants and researchers) understandings collaboratively.

Data generation and analysis

Stringer's (1999) cycle of looking, thinking and acting guided the approach used in this inquiry. Look, think and act guided every aspect of data generation and analysis incorporating one to one interviews and participatory action research group processes. *Looking* meant gathering information, defining and describing the situation. *Thinking* referred to exploring, analysing, interpreting and explaining. *Thinking* was stimulated as participants asked: 'What is happening here?' 'Why are things as they are?'

Data were generated from five sources:

(1) In-depth one to one interviews with 15 participants.
(2) Participatory action mixed gender research groups.
(3) A single page questionnaire completed by participants asking them to describe fatigue.
(4) Researcher's/facilitator's reflection and observational notes.
(5) Debrief data: the research team debriefed regularly to provide feedback for the action cycles to follow.

A multidisciplinary project management team (PMT) was convened and consulted on a regular basis and facilitated the inquiry's progress. The role of this team was to:

(1) Overview the research process and time lines.
(2) Contribute as requested to participatory action research groups when expertise was requested.
(3) Actively promote and disseminate outcome information to their agencies and beyond.
(4) In addition, the PMT was a reference point for recruitment of participants, offering individual expertise to the project, e.g. district nurses, pharmacologists, medical doctors, and critical reading of reports and subsequent publications.

Procedure

Inviting volunteers to participate in the inquiry using local newsletters and an existing network for people who were HIV 'positive' proved successful. The average age of participants was 47 years; the youngest person was 33 years and the oldest was 62 years. They had an average time living with HIV of 13.8 years, within a range of 5 to 25 years. The effect of fatigue on the people in this group was evident by their employment status. Only one participant was working full-time, eight part-time and six were on disability or old-age pensions. They all lived in urban areas in a variety of public and private housing. Of the 15 participants interviewed, two women and seven men (often joined by their partners) joined the participatory action research groups.

We invited people interested in participating in the study to contact us by telephone. An information sheet and consent form was posted out to potential participants. Sometime after, the researcher made contact to answer any questions and if the person chose to participate, a time and place was made for an interview.

At this stage each person was given the option of having the interview conducted at their home or any other mutually suitable location. Nine participants chose to be interviewed at their home, one at the research office and the remainder at various HIV community agencies.

Adequate time for engagement between participant and researcher was ensured prior to the interview. Trust of both the researcher and the research process needed to develop. The need to establish rapport was seen as important because several participants were concerned that due to past experiences with stigma, their HIV status should be kept confidential. Nevertheless, participants were keen that their stories of living with fatigue be told. Interviewing in the home helped to create a shift of influence from researcher to the participant, as it was their 'turf', in which their daily life occured, and they felt comfortable. Taped interviews lasted between 30 minutes and 2 hours.

Our aim is to where possible, involve families and/or significant others, as living with a chronic condition affects not only the person but also the people with whom he/she lives. So when relatives, partners or friends were present, time was needed to ensure that the participant was comfortable with their presence and that the research process, aims and objectives were clear to them. Three partners or family members took up the invitation to stay and gave their version of the ways that fatigue had intruded upon their lives.

Prior to the commencement of the interview a number of important issues were discussed with the participant, all of which were also clearly set out on the consent form. Issues of confidentiality were discussed at length, in addition to how the research team would use the information generated during the research. Participants were given the option of withdrawing from the inquiry at any stage or they could refrain from answering questions. Participants were made aware that they would not be identified by name and that they were able to stop the tape at any time. All names are fictional and any significant details that may have identified the participant have been changed or suppressed, while keeping the integrity of the story, to promote confidentiality.

Interviews were recorded using a small tape recorder with a discreet tabletop active microphone to improve the sound coverage. Interviewing in a person's home does not give the same controlled environment as an office and there were times when frequent low flying planes or a neighbour's lawn mower competed. One office interview was interrupted by staff coming in uninvited, and a fire alarm was heard in another wing of the building.

Several participants had previously been involved in research studies, primarily quantitative type studies related to medication trials. It was therefore necessary to provide a brief explanation of the difference between qualitative research and quantitative research.

Talking the participant through what they should expect from our interview and our rationale for gathering storied accounts of living with fatigue was appreciated.

Questions guiding the interview

The participatory action research methodology provides for the agenda to be collaboratively set by the participant and the researcher. Participants were asked to describe their experience of living with fatigue in whatever way they chose (look). They were invited to reflect on (think about) their fatigue experiences and then they were asked about ways in which they manage fatigue (act) (Box 4.1). Silences were expected and acknowledged. Moments of silence are interpreted as encouraging participants to think more clearly about their situation before responding. Questions related to gaining an understanding of fatigue, subjective responses to fatigue, contextual descriptions of when fatigue occurs and participant interpretations or 'sense-making' of the overall experience of fatigue.

During the interview the interviewer was occasionally asked clinical/ medical questions about fatigue as well as other health issues. These were answered as the interview progressed or left, if possible, to the end of the interview once the tape recorder was switched off. An

---

Box 4.1   Participatory action research interview questions.

- Demographic information
  — Age and date of birth

- Would you please tell me your story?
  — History of HIV, including approximate date of diagnosis
  — Current health status, including viral load and CD4 counts
  — Co-morbidities, if any

- What does fatigue mean to you?
  — What about before you had HIV?

- Can you describe what fatigue is like for you?
  — Today
  — Normally
  — Tell me about an example of when fatigue was too much for you

- How does fatigue affect what you do every day?

- How do you manage fatigue?
  — Who or what helps you manage?
  — Who or what hinders your ability to manage?

undertaking was made to put the person in contact with someone who could help him or her.

Interviewer's reflective notes

Immediately upon leaving the house and returning to the office, the researcher wrote fieldnotes about his impressions of the interview, descriptive data of the surroundings, body language and affect on the participant, and any other pertinent data that might help the research team understand the context. Reflection is about learning to understand our human situation and ourselves as we try to construe meaning in experiences and situations of which we are a part. As researchers, we are the instruments through which the research process is facilitated. Through reflection we learn about ourselves. It is reflection that allows us to fine-tune our skills and understanding, and thus profit from our experiences.

A reflective process and its analysis means that the researcher reflects on the role of the researcher and considers what could have happened differently; what went well, and more importantly, identify the prompts or questions that facilitated story telling. In so doing, during subsequent interviews the researcher can subtly change his/her strategies of establishing rapport, managing silences in conversations, and encouraging themes to develop, as well as adding to the analytical process of the data.

Individual interviews

The steps we are about to describe are useful for novice researchers. During this research, community nursing clinicians were being mentored during the data generation and analysis phases, so it was important to provide clear guidelines. The approach to interviewing that we have presented here has the underlying assumption that people as authors of their own lives have gathered understandings during their journeys, experiences and life events. We take their views of the world, their records, perceptions and descriptions of events as being legitimate. Stringer & Genat (2004, p. 34) proposed that the intent of interviewing:

> '. . . is not to convince [people] of the inadequacies of their perspective, but to find ways of enabling them, through sharing each other's perspectives, to formulate more productive understandings of their own situation.'

The challenge for us as the researchers is to create the opportunity for reflective conversations. To do so, we need to be sensitive to create a context that is conducive to rich interaction, to come to know each person before reflective conversations can take place. For many participants engaged in the participatory action research process, reflection begins with experiencing doubt about their interpretation of their experiences. People may doubt what seemed obvious in their lives. Experiencing doubt about one's world can be highly threatening. Certainly for some participants, reflecting on past experiences can be an uncomfortable process.

Assuming that this is the first interview with the person, the same question(s) are asked although not always in the same order. When the participant's 'story' unfolds some question(s) may be answered, so active, attentive listening is important. Often the person being interviewed will ascertain whether you are really interested in their story and if affirmative, feel enticed to respond in paragraphs rather than short responses. Generating a story line with the person means that you are interested in what the participant has to say, so direct questions are avoided. Sometimes finding the place to start a story can be difficult and the participant may 'hesitate' a few times as they consciously try to order or sequence the events that have been important to them. Allow the person the time and space to sort through their story and for it to emerge. The interview process is dialogical but your voice should be minimal in this dialogical process. Prompts used sensitively can stimulate conversation:

- Tell me more about . . . ?
- How did that make you feel?
- I don't quite understand; can you explain further?
- What do you mean by . . . ?
- What matters to you?
- What is important to you?

Guided by the look, think and act process:

- Let us look at this again; what . . . ?
- Let us think about what you have said; what . . . ?
- What sort of actions do you envisage could result from this . . . ?

A research journal is maintained. These interviewer's notes record the context and show what happened whilst generating data. Reflection on the interview episode is carried out by asking: What worked well and what can be done differently? Subsequent interviews become more skilled as an outcome of these reflections.

During this inquiry, three questions were asked of all participants. This structure assists novice researchers to begin analysis confidently as these questions can shape the analysis. The questions were: What is fatigue? What constitutes self-management of fatigue? What are the constraints and enablers to self-management? The term 'self-management' makes reference to the activities people undertake to create order, discipline and control in their lives (Kralik et al., 2004). The framework provided below can guide data analysis. Missing from this analysis framework is the context in which these stories take hold. Rather, the framework can lead to an analysis of experience, from which a co-constructed storyline might be developed.

Story telling: analysis protocol

The analysis can be shaped by the nature and sequence of questions asked. When a participant is asked to tell his/her story with few structured questions, the analysis protocol provided below could be useful. This protocol includes strategies for analysing multiple stories to create a single story line.

Story making is a cyclical process. In the example given we interview each person individually, the transcript is analysed and a story line is formulated by the researcher. This story line is returned to the person whose story it is and shared with co-researchers. Once all stakeholders have read and made changes, we argue that the final story line has been co-constructed and validated by all stakeholders. Co-construction of the story line makes visible the way ongoing concerns play out in everyday practice to produce coherent selves and construct diversity and difference.

Step 1. Read through the entire transcript to get the sense of the whole

- Read through the transcripts with an 'attunement' to both the content of the words, how their selection and combination represent the particular voice(s) of the participants, including those who speak and those they speak about, and what the words mean in relation to the actual experiences of the participants.
- Read each transcript several times to gain further familiarity with the words, the voices they represent, the meanings they hold for the speaker and the order in which they had been spoken.
- In doing so, try to 'engage' with the words of the participant by reflecting on the fact that their words and how they are combined in the language of the transcript represent participants' own choices on how to render their experience. In engaging with their stories, then, remember that you are interpreting the choices they have made.

Step 2. With the transcript in front of you commence analysis of the data

- First level of clustering. Cluster (group) responses (data) to answer interview questions (e.g. What is fatigue? How do you manage it and what are the constraints to management? What really matters?). Group these into paragraphs.

- Second level of clustering. You will notice that the participant has chosen not only to answer the few questions you have posed in their own unique style, but also other aspects of their experiences are revealed. These need to be grouped separately. Look for similar experiences or ideas so that you can cluster/group these data together in one paragraph. Look, think and act questions/answers can assist with shaping this analysis. Ask what is going on (look), what is being reflected on here (think) and what action is proposed (act). Place data into separate paragraphs under look, think and act to help shape the analysis.

- Third level. What really matters? It is important to group these data under this heading.

- Fourth level. In reading the above paragraphs, what do you think is happening here or what is significant?

- You have grouped the data into the questions/responses, into other aspects of the participant's experiences, into what matters, and you have asked what is significant in each of these paragraphs. Now determine the significant statements.

Step 3. Determine the significant statements (see example extracting significant statement from Albert Baker's story, Appendix 1)

- Identify significant statements expressed by the participant and rewrite paragraphs with the most significant statement at the helm.

- Ask: What does this significant statement tell me about what it is like to live with ... ? What makes this statement significant?

- Repeat this question for each of the significant statements. List all significant statements (this list will be used for subsequent interview analysis).

- Describe, in a clear, simple manner, what you think is going on to make this statement significant.

(1) Using a significant statement as the first sentence of the paragraph write one paragraph about that person's experience in your own words.

(2) It is important to ensure that each paragraph explores one significant aspect or experience.

(3) Each paragraph should begin with a significant statement (the first sentence of the paragraph).

(4) Voice the text; weave one to two 'good' quotes into each paragraph. A good quote is one that captures the speaker's experience from her/his point of view.

Step 4. Writing the story

- Order the paragraphs into a story line.
- Each story illustrates an economy of style (no more than two pages of single space text for each story). This story is often incorporated into a resource complied with participants, or the final report or subsequent publications, hence the need for economy of style.

Step 5. Reading and sharing the story with the research team

- Read the story for cohesiveness, engagement and whether it answers the questions posed. Imagine that you are a reader who has never met or talked with the participant. Does the story communicate their experience and values?
- If research is conducted in a team, colleagues are asked to read the story and provide critical comment.
- Researchers analyse each transcript separately and then work collaboratively in recreating the individual story line.
- The story is then given to the participant for further co-construction.

Step 6. Reading and co-constructing the story with the participant (see Chester's story below)

- The story can be built (co-constructed) using the significant statements and paragraphs subsumed under the heading of the research question asked. The participant is given the story and is asked to review the story line and make changes.
- Co-construction of the story line makes visible the way ongoing concerns play out in everyday practice to both produce coherent selves and construct diversity and difference. The final story is a co-construction between researcher and participant.
- Validation of the story enhances methodological rigour.

Step 7. Combining participants' stories into one common story line. Individual interview analysis processes and story writing are repeated for each transcript

- Compile a list of all significant statements from each of the stories (see 3.3); that is, list all significant statements (those statements you have used to start each sentence and recorded).
- Identify the source of each statement (where we can locate the entire paragraph and statement). Write the common story line.

Appendix 1, Albert Baker's story, will show the way in which significant statements were extracted. To provide an example, in following section we will share Chester's individual story.

Chester's story

Chester was in a long term relationship and confidently stated that he has been HIV-positive since 1978, when he had a profound sero-conversion reaction. He identified fatigue as something that has been with him throughout his life but exacerbated since contracting HIV. He retired from work 20 years ago in a concerted effort to manage his fatigue symptoms. He has a level of self-agency in his management of fatigue that is a result of self-awareness and self-confidence to make decisions that positively affect his life. Central to this effort was his wish that:

'I want to have a high quality life. I want to enjoy when I'm awake fully . . . I don't want to feel exhausted all the time.'

What is fatigue?

Fatigue was a part of Chester's life, requiring him to develop strategies to rest well, before HIV also became part of his life. He described relishing sleep as a child until boarding school took away that opportunity.

Chester suggested that there is a subtle pressure to deny fatigue is an issue in our society. Similarly to depression, talking about fatigue isn't something that is acceptable or tolerated in society. Stoicism and a strong work ethic is the acceptable response in our society, which presents difficulties when fatigue is present in your life.

Chester felt that fatigue had aged him prematurely, especially in terms of his self-concept. He talks of being 'old-aged' when he feels fatigued and having to learn the habits of old age.

Fatigue as a symptom of HIV is not constant in its severity. Rather, Chester describes it as cyclical or episodic, varying from moment to moment:

'Had we been having this interview in six months hence or six months ago or some other time, my answers might be completely different, completely different . . . When it's more, it affects my everyday life in every way. When it's less, it's just a manageable thing I suppose.'

Episodes of HIV treatment have exacerbated fatigue, whether due to the therapy itself or the physical effort of having to travel to and from hospital:

'Fatigue is defined as "tired weakness" in a physical and emotional sense . . . if you're already in bed and you're flat on your back, you think it's just my muscles won't let me get up, my mind won't let me get up because I just can't, that's what it feels like. And if you're already walking or doing something, it's just well I just can't do this any longer, I need to stop.'

Depression is not directly linked to fatigue symptoms for Chester. He can be fatigued without a depressed affect:

'I think depression and fatigue are sort of linked but not causally, they're just coincidentally linked I think.'

Some medications can add to fatigue. Antidepressants, which Chester has taken for analgesic effect rather than for depression, have had the effect of giving him an over-confidence in his abilities to do tasks, with the end result being even more fatigue than at the start.

How is fatigue managed?

Awareness of fatigue is the first step to successfully managing it. Chester said:

'I think the most important message is to pay attention to the symptoms of fatigue . . . I've learned to recognize it.'

Self-management of fatigue revolves around Chester giving himself permission to relax, rest and make personal decisions in life that facilitate this. Chester gave himself permission to give priority to his needs. This is evidenced by his decision to retire and change some of his daily work practices. However, he understands the enormity of such a change and recognises that not everyone is lucky enough to have this ability:

'That's a very big step, so if we were talking about that, you know, that working mother with two mortgages and two children and two jobs, who's got HIV, then she suffers fatigue, experiencing fatigue or other symptoms, then she's got the problem giving herself permission, I don't. I just sometimes feel guilty about not getting up early enough to feed the chooks, but now D does that, so I don't even have to worry about that!'

Making these changes entailed a process of learning for Chester. He had to teach himself to 'slow down':

'Just pacing myself, just managing it, re-learning, you know, just saying this doesn't have to be done today, you know, this doesn't have to be done, you can put your feet up.'

Sleep is a significant management strategy, not only in response to feeling fatigued but as a pre-emptive measure. Chester recognized this very early in his life and made sure that he created opportunities for sleep and rest where possible. His work situation allowed him to do this but at a personal cost:

'... when I was busy, I would get a phone book or two and put them behind my desk, out of sight on the floor and nap, every lunchtime almost without fail and the switchboard knew it, when I didn't have ... lunch and my co-workers knew it ... But they thought it was eccentric, now that's 20 years ago and I don't think people think that's eccentric now.'

Chester suggests that all workplaces have areas for employees to rest without prejudice. He is certain that this would increase productivity.

Chester avoids alcohol but uses marijuana. He did not state what effect this has for him or the intent when it is used. Chester appears to have reached a level of self-agency that allows him to live a life that, while still limited, enables him to enjoy himself.

Preparation for the participatory action research group process

Chester was given his story with an invitation to read and amend it and return it to the researchers. In this way the story was co-constructed. He was also asked to sign a consent form for it to be used in the research report and any subsequent publications.

When one to one interviews were concluded and each participant had received his or her story, it was then the task of the research team to compile a composite document for discussion at participatory action research groups. In preparation for participatory action research groups, a document comprising 15 stories and a summary of major themes was posted to all participants. Participants reportedly liked receiving their stories and felt validated by the process. Very few changes were made, with most being dates of diagnosis, medication names and the like. Major themes remained unchanged in all stories.

Participatory action research groups

Following Stringer's (1999) participatory action research principles, which favour consensual and participatory procedures, participants were enabled to set the agenda for discussion, to prioritize issues they wished to discuss and devise plans to deal with the issues at hand.

During the initial contact with people interested in participating in the research project, it was made clear that there would not only be face to face interviews but also the opportunity to meet as a group to share stories and discuss fatigue self-management.

When one to one interviews had been completed, time was spent describing the participatory action research process and inviting the participant to attend participatory action research groups. This was described so that it was clear they would have the opportunity to learn more about fatigue and its management from HIV specialists and other people who lived with fatigue, as well as an opportunity to tell their own stories and take individual or collaborative action.

Of the fifteen interviewed, nine participants (two women and seven men) took part in these meetings. Six participants attended both meetings, one attended only the first and two were able to only come to the second meeting. Five participants attended with friends, family or partners.

Taxi transport was offered to those for whom transport would be an issue. Childcare was offered to both women who had young children, and was used by one woman for both meetings.

A healthy choices dinner was provided, which included a choice of cold and hot food and refreshments. The sharing of a meal facilitated casual conversation between participants, which was important to reduce the anxiety associated with speaking out in a group situation. The mixed gender group, along with partners/friends, spent a total of 5 hours together, excluding the meal breaks.

Preparation prior to convening participatory action research groups

There were a number of important issues to consider before the meetings: numbers, timing, location, partners/friends and seating.

Numbers

We have found that the ideal number of people for a group session such as this is between eight and twelve. This gives people the chance to have their say without being swamped by the conversations of others. If there are less than eight participants, then people may feel vulnerable and thus less willing to speak about their experiences.

Timing

We invited the participants and partners/friends to attend on weekday nights between 17.30 and 20.00. This time was chosen to allow those participants who were working to have the opportunity to attend while recognizing that having fatigue often diminishes the ability to stay out late at night. The time frame gave enough time for introductions and housekeeping, an informal meal and an opportunity to talk to clinical specialists if people desired.

Location

The meetings were held at a central location, with easy parking, access to toilets and catering facilities.

Partners and friends

The ability to bring a partner or friend increased the number of participants joining the participatory action research group. Some participants found moral support in having someone with them, while some relied on others to share their interpretations of stories. As discussed previously, the impact of living with a chronic illness intrudes not only on the person but also his/her partner, so it was important that the voices of significant others were included. Partners and friends were encouraged to participate and contribute to the discussions.

Seating

To ensure that all present felt equal in their ability to participate in discussions, seating for the group was arranged in an open circular inward-facing format. Nearby, but out of the circle, was the table where conversations were transcribed verbatim by the clerical person, using a laptop computer. A chair was placed in the centre to accommodate the tape recorder and microphone. An effort was made to ensure that each participant could see everyone else. Researchers positioned themselves interspersed throughout the group to lessen any foci of power.

The story line is communicated to participatory action research group participants

In the analysis process each story responded to statements such as: What is fatigue? How is fatigue self-managed? These significant statements shaped the core of the common story line. Some participants told of abject frustration with fatigue that consumed large portions of their lives. Other participants reported fatigue side-effects resulting from medical treatments. A few participants had co-morbid medical conditions, such as hepatitis or cancer, that complicated their assessment of fatigue. Age and life experiences varied widely. The majority of participants, 13 men, contracted HIV from homosexual transmission, whilst the two women had contracted HIV from intravenous drug use.

Despite this diversity, there was a common thread running through these stories. Participants all experienced fatigue. Fatigue is something that is or is being incorporated into the lives of these people and there were common goals of minimizing its intrusion. What they report are sophisticated yet often simple self-management strategies that manipulate the environment as well as the self. Manipulating work and rest times sounds simple but can present endless complicating obstacles when one is trying to keep a job, raise children or have a pleasurable social life. Pushing the boundaries is something that needs to occur to facilitate this happening. This can mean that a consequence is mental or physical exertion past the point of exhaustion, knowing the impact the following day will be significant. Perhaps this might mean staying out later at a social engagement, as time with friends or family is valued and enjoyable, despite knowing that during the days to follow there will be little to offer in terms of energy.

At the first participatory action research session

The common story line was sent to each participant prior to participatory action research group meetings. At the beginning of each participatory action research group, introductions and group norms were established.

Introductions

'Breaking the ice'. All present were invited to introduce themselves to the group. Introductions were recorded so that we could hear the way in which participants choose to share aspects of their self-identity. Researchers gave context to their roles in the inquiry. Participants spoke briefly about their history of HIV and fatigue. Introductions were done before the evening meal to maximize conversation and rapport building.

Group norms

Following the principles of participatory action research, participants were encouraged to contribute their thoughts on what the group norms (rules as some put it) should be for the sessions. Ownership of these by the group encouraged them to take the process more seriously than if a list had simply been presented to them by the facilitator. It gave an early indication that this was their group and they were able to set the agenda. Norms suggested by the participants were confidentiality, giving each other the opportunity to share their stories with equal 'air-space' and to advocate only one person speaking at a time.

At the first session, participants and researchers discussed the composite story line document that had been distributed by mail.

The research team

Each member of the research team had key roles to play in the participatory action research group:

- The project manager facilitated the participatory action research groups because he had been present during all of the interviews; the participants saw him as a familiar face. He also conducted the introductions, housekeeping and other initial discussions as a way of 'breaking the ice' and making participants feel comfortable with the process. He presented the common story line to the participatory action research group.
- The first author co-facilitated the participatory action research process.
- Clinical nurse consultants (CNCs) attended meetings to provide clinical information as needed. Interestingly, there was little if any call for this as the participants clearly were a well-informed group who had a clear understanding of the physical and social issues, particularly about HIV and partly about fatigue.
- The research administrator organized catering and name badges, and entered real time verbatim transcripts of the group discussions onto a laptop computer.

This mix of researchers and health professionals provided a comprehensive view of the process and at the same time provided for education and support. The participants were clearly well informed and articulate about HIV and fatigue, as well as the contextual issues that affected living with these. The HIV clinicians remarked about how little information they had needed to add to the discussion.

Transcription of dialogue

Recording and typing conversations in real time is an exhausting but rigorous process. Skilled, fast typing results in immediate access to data once the group has dissipated. In the transcript of these conversations it is easy to see who was speaking. While participatory action research conversations are taking place, researchers can observe and record descriptions of actions and body language. Verbatim transcripts were available immediately following each session. Analysis was able to occur with the events fresh in the minds of those present. In accord with the cyclical nature of sessions and feedback to participants, issues and concerns could be brought back to the group the following week for clarification. One of the group norms established at the beginning of each session was to have only one person speaking at a time. This was not only a measure of courtesy to each other but also made transcription much easier. It was also very important to ensure that breaks were scheduled at least hourly to give the word processing person a break from typing 100+ words per minute. Clearly the skills of speed typing are essential here.

Group facilitation

The facilitators play an important role in the participatory action research process. Managing the dynamics of the group included: facilitating any cross-cultural sensitivities, promoting feelings of equality for all people involved; maintaining harmony; avoiding conflicts; resolving conflicts that arise; encouraging personal, cooperative relationships rather than impersonal, competitive, conflicting or authoritarian relationships; and being sensitive to people's feelings. These sensitivities were discussed at the commencement of the first group with participants, and were identified as 'group norms'.

Intrinsic to the participatory action research approach is that the participants' issues and agendas are at the centre of the research process. The participants own the agenda and this ultimately leads to them taking charge of the participatory action process and the outcome. As with all group work, individual personalities make the process unpredictable and there are always some instances where participants take the conversations in obscure directions. Nevertheless, the facilitator attempts to refrain from re-directing the conversations. One of the most difficult tasks for researchers new to the participatory action research process is to relax and trust the process, letting people decide the direction of the conversations. In our experiences, group members usually self-regulate. When a conversation has gone on for too long, other participants usually remind everyone that each person present should have a turn to talk. The relaxed approach taken by the facilitator avoids the desire to be in control of group processes.

Facilitators need to be sensitive, to create a context that is conducive to rich interaction, to come to know each person before reflective conversations can take place. Too much threat and participants may become overwhelmed and withdraw from the process. Too much safety and they may not be challenged sufficiently to take the leap into reflecting on their experiences. A participant reflected on the experience of this balance:

> 'It has been a learning and discovery time, time to reflect, time to make changes and like others in the study it has allowed plenty of debriefing and growth.'

Facilitation involves assisting individuals and the group as a whole to talk about their experiences of living with fatigue and identify successes and barriers they have faced along the way. At the same time there was the chance to discuss and begin to develop new management techniques, seek information from the HIV specialist in the group (rarely), and engage in group issue-solving and individual decision-making. The research team collaborated to provide individuals with the basis for beginning to make self-management choices and achieving self-selected goals. In this way, participants were facilitated to consider new or different ways to incorporate their condition into their lives.

The process of look, think and act framed the discussions, and validation of the story line document that had been previously distributed as well as the summary of the previous meeting's discussion meant that activity spiralled. Participatory action research groups identified issues of importance on which they felt strongly enough to take action.

Debriefing

When each meeting had finished and the participants had left, the research team met to share their reflections and feelings about the session. Notes of this debriefing were taken and made available to those researchers undertaking analysis to ensure the context of the participatory action research process was enhanced. As a preliminary analysis procedure, the research team met to decide on the main themes and decide on feedback to be given to participants at the next meeting. This is usually referred to as the cyclic feedback loop in the participatory action research process.

Data analysis and feedback

Data analysis involves the identification of prominent features within a data set. In this research, data from participatory action research sessions were analysed concurrently. Together we generated 37 pages of transcribed text. The analysis process for participatory action research dialogues follows five steps.

Step 1. Read through the entire transcript

- Read through the transcripts with an 'attunement' to both the content of the words and the actual experiences of the participants.
- Read each transcript several times to gain further familiarity with the words and the order in which they had been spoken.
- Identify group dynamics and power play and ways in which these affect data generation.
- Share the above deliberations with the research team for further discussion and elaboration prior to the next cycle.

Step 2. Cluster dialogue under look, think and act framework

- The research questions were: What is fatigue? What is your experience of fatigue? What are the constraints to self-management? A common story line was presented to each participant and discussed in the participatory action research groups.
- Analysis structure is provided by look, think and act.
- Look: What does the group have to say about fatigue?
- Think: What does the group think they might be able to do to change or improve the situation?
- Act: What kind of actions may result?
- Identify main themes.

Step 3. Cycle: provide feedback on the main themes under the look, think and act structure

- Articulate the main themes emerging from the data.
- Order the paragraphs into a story line outlining what the group thinks, what the group has reflected on, and what it intends to do.
- Record and monitor look, think and act themes through subsequent cycles.
- Alter the story line as new themes emerge (co-construction).

Step 4. Collaboratively decide and plan action

- Co-construction of the story line makes visible the way ongoing concerns play out in everyday life.
- A composite story is a co-construction between researcher and participant.
- Validation of the story enhances methodological rigour.

Step 5. Facilitate and record actions

- What has changed?
- How will these changes be sustained?

Data analysis is often enhanced by incorporating non-interview data, such as journals, researchers' observational notes, and information already gleaned from the literature. There is often existing research that will help to frame or challenge commonly held assumptions held by health workers and community members.

Feedback cycles

It is vitally important that findings are brought back to the group for discussion and validation. This is often referred to as cycles of information and feedback. Validation of findings, usually concurrently, is a requirement of working with people in the process of participatory action research. Alan praised this process:

> 'Impressive to me is the to and fro process, you coming back to us and refining, that really makes me feel appreciated and useful. Not just telling us and go away and you'll never hear from us again.'

Validation occurs when participants are given the findings from the previous session at the start of the next meeting. This is again part of the cyclic feedback loop crucial in the participatory action research process. In this way, data are generated with participants, new understandings emerge and findings are congruent with participants' experiences of living with fatigue.

Subsequent participatory action research group meetings commenced with discussion of the main themes from the previous week. As group meetings progress, distinctive features and common themes from each group meeting are preserved. Theme analysis helped to shape both the content and the process of the self-management strategies put forward.

Action (individual and group level)

Participants, in collaboration with researchers, explored ways in which fatigue impacted upon their lives. *Acting* referred to the development of plans devised by participants, their implementation and evaluation. For example, a participant planned to incorporate alternative strategies into the day-to-day management of fatigue and then took action to implement that plan. The participant then reported back to the group the outcome of those actions.

Whilst it is not possible to present the entire study, it is relevant to share some of the actions generated by people participating in this research. In the participatory action research process used with participants who live with fatigue, the action component of the process refers to changing or adapting 'self' management strategies and taking action in one's own life. Individuals decide to incorporate some of the strategies they have learned from others in the group (other participants, facilitator and educator) into their self-management.

Occasionally participatory action research results in action from the group as a whole as they make an attempt to reform the world around them. This group of participants was of the strong opinion that the information they had generated with the research team needed to be shared with as many people as possible. We had already explained that their stories would be used in an article that would be submitted to a refereed journal to inform other health care professionals. As well, there was a mutual wish that the resultant report be circulated to selected government and non-government agencies that provided services to people with chronic illness and HIV in particular. Some of this was in response to the continued stigma that HIV generated, which obscured understanding. Chester summed it up eloquently:

> 'I would like to have a letter to the Archbishops and these other groups. It seems to be the churches are a big player in setting the acceptance agenda. Other groups like Rotary, Lions, Legacy . . . haven't been involved at all. These groups do good work to include us. The stigma of fatigue is pervasive and it needs to be understood that they aren't just too tired; they can't cut their firewood, cut their own lawns. [Tuberculosis] was associated with sexual looseness years ago, women got it. Men didn't. It's HIV now and we have to get beyond this stigma.'

It was suggested by the research team and agreed by participants that an executive summary of the report be distributed to various agencies determined by the group. It was agreed that readers would be invited to access the full report on the research unit web site if they wished (www.rdns.net.au).

The group suggested that the findings of this research project be presented at the next National Association of People with HIV/AIDS (NAPWA) Conference. In addition, it was suggested that Relationships Australia run a forum where research findings are communicated to service providers who would not necessarily have the ability to access conference proceedings.

An appeal was made to unite and draft a letter to state and federal parliamentary ministers responsible for local government and the HACC scheme, to voice concern about the inequity and lack of uniformity between different agencies that provided or should provide services to HIV-positive people living with fatigue. Two participants told the group that they are already on a working party of People Living with HIV/Aids (SA Inc.) and these matters were being progressed. They offered their services to formulate an advocacy letter for all participants to sign.

Centrelink, a South Australian government agency that provides financial benefits to the majority of the participants, also received attention from the PAR group. It was suggested that this key government organization needed to make up a training kit that educates workers about the complexity of fatigue in HIV and other chronic illnesses. This was in response to issues participants had had in assessments for different benefits that did not take into account on the day of assessment, the fluctuating nature of fatigue.

Evaluation and sustainability

Process evaluation was conducted by asking participants during the final participatory action research meeting to comment on the research process as a whole, including the interviews and group sessions. In addition, Kenneth was appreciative of the chance to use the questionnaire as a catalyst for a discussion with his partner about fatigue and how it affected both of them:

> 'I think it's been quite an experience and interesting to hear the stories that relate to fatigue, I think that's probably the most interesting part for me. I'd written those two questions, myself and my partner went quite deeply into those. I didn't want to repeat my story so we had a think together and he told me his side, what he noticed about me, so there is a reasonable amount of information in that. That's about all I can say. But I'm keen to meet again in the group.'

Participants have indicated that they wish to continue meeting with each other. One desirable outcome of the participatory action research process is that it can be sustained without facilitation.

In this chapter we have shown what happens when we work *with* people who live with a chronic condition, in this case HIV and fatigue. We have discussed the many components of the participatory action research application that are required to ensure the best outcomes: setting, education, facilitation, story telling, sharing, action and sustainability. The potential for action at an individual and group level was highlighted and specific examples have been given.

5 Learning to Learn

In this chapter we share our understanding of the participatory action process and principles for use in the community. What happens when we learn in a participatory action process? We discuss and illustrate the processes of group interaction and learning. As discussed earlier, we are guided by the participants in our efforts to reshape our health practice. Listening and learning are core activities in participatory action research practice because it is a process where the focus is on learning to be in this world with all the capacities we have.

Learning

In the following section we share some dialogue to show the way in which learning can occur within a participatory action research group.

One participatory action research inquiry (Koch et al., 2003) responded to the high prevalence of older people living in the community with asthma (Box 5.1). The principle aim for this inquiry was to develop,

---

Box 5.1   A summary of the study by Koch et al. (2003) as conveyed in the *Journal of Evidence-Based Nursing*.

Participants
Twenty-four community dwelling adults >60 years of age (67% women, mean age 76 years, age range 60–92 years) with medically diagnosed asthma who were using, or had been prescribed, daily preventative medications.

Methods
Data were collected using one to one in-depth interviews, an open ended questionnaire, and two mixed gender participatory action research groups. In-depth interviews lasting about 1 hour each were held in the participants' homes and guiding questions were used to help participants reflect on their personal asthma self-management story. Interviews were tape

---

(Continued)

Box 5.1   *(Continued).*

recorded, transcribed verbatim and collaboratively analysed by three researchers. Eighteen participants and six invited partners participated in two participatory action research meetings to collaboratively develop a model that would enable self-management of asthma for older people. Participatory action research meetings were transcribed and analysed concurrently to ensure prompt feedback of issues to participants. The voices of participants were represented in the text to enhance study rigour. In addition to ongoing feedback as part of the participatory action research cycle, the study report was validated by all participants.

Main findings

Three models of asthma management emerged: a medical model, a collaborative model, and a self-agency model. Most participants described being in a medical model of asthma management. In this model, the key to self-management was taking prescribed medications, which the participants mostly took the responsibility of managing themselves. Participants also identified and avoided triggers for asthma attacks. In this model, the doctor managed the disease process and the participants trusted and followed the doctor's authority. The doctor's authority, however, was more likely to be trusted if the doctor provided specific disease knowledge and sound medical advice.

Some participants described a collaborative model of asthma management in which asthma self-management involved other people, or was perceived by participants to be their own agency. Collaborative management was most likely to be a joint effort between participants and health care professionals. Participants were not only offered medical advice, but also had input into the decision making process regarding their care. When participant input was acknowledged and valued, it was conducive to self-agency in the asthma management process.

The self-agency model of asthma management involved self-identification of responses to illness and the self-planning of daily routines to create order in daily life. Taking control of their own lives was an important part of self-management, and taking action with daily life routines facilitated self-determination. Participants who described using a self-agency model talked about self-management only in terms of their own agency. They took control of their own illness and responses to illness, and decided when to share their management decisions with their doctor.

Conclusions

In community living, older adults with asthma described three models of asthma self-management: the medical, collaborative, and self-agency models. Participants described self-management as reclaiming the self and regaining self-identity, including achieving recognition and support for the self-monitoring process.

Reproduced with permission of the BMJ Publishing Group, from *Evidence-Based Nursing* (2005) **8**, 127.

in collaboration with older people, a client-led model of asthma
management that acknowledged the context of an individual's life.
The secondary aim was that the participatory action research group
sustained the model after the researchers had left 'the field' and that
it was transferable to other settings. The objectives were:

(1)   To understand from the perspective of older men and women
      living with asthma how the illness has impacted on their lives.
(2)   To identify the contexts, barriers and issues that are significant for
      older people living with asthma.
(3)   In collaboration with the participants, to design, implement and
      evaluate an asthma self-management model.
(4)   To develop a sustainable and replicable model which facilitates
      self-management for older people living with asthma.

Getting started

A group of older people were brought together, shared lunch and
commenced a facilitated 3-hour dialogue. In the first group session with
12 people, including researchers and one asthma educator, Finlay,
who was aged 90, shared his story with the group:

> 'My name is Finlay and I understand I had asthma at two years of age.
> My mum took me for a walk in the pram and it was a cold and rainy day,
> she didn't care for me as I expected, and that's how I finished with asthma.
> When I was 12 I rode a bicycle, it was recommended to help the lungs.
> That didn't happen. I rode for some years and various treatments were tried
> when trying to find help; I even went to the gas works in Sydney to inhale
> the gas off the road-tarring process. That used to be tried in those days.
> I don't know if I benefited or not. Ipecac wine was another thing they used
> to use. Asthma came back on me when I was 40. I have had various treat-
> ments since, being at the asthma clinic, the doctor's rooms that have helped
> me. I was using Pulmicort as an inhaler – a preventative. It was so irritat-
> ing on my throat I couldn't talk. I haven't taken Pulmicort for about 12 months
> on a regular basis but before that I was hoarse and it was difficult to hear
> what I was saying. I don't want to repeat that with Flixatide. I was faithful
> in washing the mouth out and gargling. When I feel discomfort I resort to
> the Ventolin. It's almost instant – I carry it with me wherever I go.'

When participants first share stories they tend to focus on symptoms
and therapies. When everyone in the group had had a chance to share
their story it was usual for people's stories to evolve in subsequent meetings to include not only their medical situation but also the contexts
in which their lives are lived. As Finlay's introductory excerpt shows,
his storied account started with his medical diagnosis, the duration of
the chronic illness and current medications, but eventually we heard

about the impact this condition had on his everyday life. When people become better acquainted, greater risks are taken in sharing and divulging experiences and the group begins to appreciate the diversity in people's management strategies. The group learns together the way in which this condition can be managed differently.

As stories are exchanged, group interaction and learning from each other should not be underestimated. This is what Megan had to say to Finlay:

'Flixatide might have extra "oomph" in it, but it is a cortisone type thing, therefore you are going to get thrush in the mouth and throat. It's difficult to clear up so you must rinse your mouth out and gargle. For goodness sake don't stop using it because of getting a husky voice! Your lungs are more important. It will help control the inflammation in your lungs.'

Sharing information is vitally important in the participatory action research groups. People learn from each other in the group and sometimes take advice from others into their self-care.

Sharing information

People share with the group the ways they have learned to successfully manage their condition. They are justly proud of their strengths. Even so, management strategies shared by others in the group are often incorporated into their own lives as actions at an individual level. The educator and facilitator rarely interfere with the decisions made by group members. They intervene only when the management strategy suggested has the potential to harm. Sharing occurs when participants collaboratively work towards developing chronic illness management strategies.

Returning our attention to Finlay's introductory statement, participants shared the symptom of voice loss. Julie described the symptom and the ways she is now managing it:

'I take this Ventolin – it affects my throat. Some drugs were stopping me from talking properly. My voice level has gone down. I went to a speech therapist because my voice was going. She was very expensive let me tell you. She said there is not a great deal I could do about it except change my puffers. Some puffers affect my throat badly. I have to make sure I wash the back of my throat. I have two puffers in the morning and two at night and that gave me a sore throat and thrush. I have a good excuse to have a cup of tea afterwards. And I've got a big spacer and find the cup of tea finishes me off. Maybe it's to do with the warmth.'

Jenny described the effect of oxygen (without humidification) on the voice:

'When in hospital for seven weeks on oxygen I lost my voice completely. I had to learn to speak again with a speech therapist. It had dried out my vocal chords – I had to learn to speak again, do all these exercises. I was using my false vocal chords – they put tubes up your nose and you had to make funny noises. I have to ask for humidified oxygen now.'

Jenny told the group about her symptom and offered advice about requesting humidified oxygen. When Jenny shared this account, participants in the group recognized that Jenny's asthma was severe, and those people in the group with mild asthma made comparisons. Linda confided to the group: 'I still feel my asthma is extremely mild and I'm thankful for that. A lot of people are much worse than I am'.

Robyn joined Linda in claiming that her asthma condition was less severe; she said: 'I'm glad to talk to other people here to see how they are managing. I'm lucky mine isn't as bad'. It is always interesting that people compare situations. We note that those who feel their asthma is mild also tend to leave the group stating that 'there are always other people worse off' (Beryl).

At the same time, participants who live with severe asthma are often proud they manage so well, taking delight in sharing their expertise and thus validating their sense of self.

Finlay considered the advice he had been offered by others in the group:

'Another point I'd make in coming here (to the participatory action group) is I've become more aware of the threats to my own health. I've not been very careful in areas suggested here, taking medication regularly. I do self-management – I think it implies that I do it. I took myself off Pulmicort and if Flixatide goes the same way I won't continue it. Ventolin is very effective to me. But coming here helps you to have a look at yourself from the viewpoint of someone outside. I learnt those two things at least and have enjoyed the information from other people.'

It is clear that Finlay is self-determining. Self-agency is implied when he states that he will take Flixatide but he will make a decision about its continuation once he has assessed the situation for himself. In medical management language Finlay would be named as non-compliant if he chose not to take Flixatide. Joining the participatory action group has given him additional information with which to make decisions about self-management.

Fear dominated the shared stories about the experiences of having an acute asthmatic attack. Naomi described the ways she overcame her fears:

'You know you're not comfortable breathing like that. Whilst doing that you think of something else, switch off from panic. I also have relaxation tapes which I put on. It is music to the sounds of the sea – very relaxing. Sometimes just relaxing in the chair with the tape on is all it needs.'

Most participants work on stress reduction or breathing exercises. Norma offered:

'I go to a yoga class, well I used to. A lot of breathing, exercise. It still must help more than hinders me. You always feel good when you come away from it.'

Jim offered the group another ways of handling breathing:

'When the chest gets tight you feel you can't breathe properly, I stand upright against a wall and force myself to take long, slow deep breaths. If it doesn't ease off then I go to the puffer.'

Penny described how she managed:

'In the cold early morning, get a wheat bag or water bottle on your chest. I like to do those quirky things before getting onto heavy things. Try simple things first.'

Others shared that breathing improved through taking hot showers and regular exercise, at which Frasier's humorous contribution was, 'Yes especially the pokies – you are pressing the buttons'.

There was a great deal of discussion around the triggers for asthma. Frasier added:

'I would suggest we are aware acutely that we are asthmatic – we need to estimate what triggers these acts – dust, preservatives in food, wine. Many other factors – some people are allergic to cats and dogs and so on. You need to take steps to avoid contact with anything that gives you problems. I think you need to try and assess and be responsible for keeping asthma under control.'

Sharing stories about triggers involved all participants and they came to realise that triggers resulted in individual responses.

A motivation for people to join participatory action research groups is the opportunity to learn from others. Just as importantly, participants like to think they are doing something that will help others. Indeed, evaluations show that participants value learning from others (those diagnosed with the same condition or symptom, such as fatigue) as one of the most significant outcomes. They envisage that action by the group has the potential to effect change in the wider world.

Being heard

In the early sessions participants were asked to share their own stories. This is often the first time people have been asked to talk about what it is like to live with a chronic illness. Being diagnosed with asthma was central to their story. This was usually followed by their responses to the illness, the impact of asthma, and how they have found a place for this chronic illness in their lives. The process of biographical work, sequencing illness events and finding meaning in their experiences of living with illness can empower participants to take action in their own lives. As each person was given the opportunity to be heard, participants learnt from the experiences of others through sharing of stories. Reflection and/or consciousness-raising usually develop among participants and they become motivated to act. In addition, the actual process of sharing stories and being 'heard' for the first time can validate their sense of self-identity. Ethical and consent issues aside, we believe that participants must be given an opportunity to read, comment, change and validate their story before it is submitted to a public arena.

Action (individual and group level)

In the participatory action research process with participants who live with asthma, the action component of the process refers to changing or adapting 'self' management strategies and people taking action in their lives. Individuals decide to take some of the strategies they have learned from others in the group (other participants, the facilitator or the educator) into their self-management. The facilitator records and monitors individual actions participants have decided upon. Individual and group responses can be traced.

Occasionally resultant action comes from the group as a whole as they make an attempt to reform the world around them. This participatory action research group instigated a strategy to send a letter to GPs and Members of Parliament asking them to support bulk billing of clients who live with asthma.

Look, think and act cycles are appealing because they can be used by research participants in their everyday lives. The appeal of this process can be attributed to its simplicity; however, a word of caution is warranted here. Asking people to reflect can be risky if recall and rethinking ignite responses of pain. Skilful facilitation is essential in the creation of a safe environment in which to talk.

During these participatory action research sessions, facilitators learn alongside participants. What is learned together is shared with others as the findings of the inquiry. At the same time the act of facilitation becomes more skilled as we appreciate group differences and dynamics. Facilitation will occupy a stand-alone chapter, which is required to do justice to the complexity of learning alongside people.

In the following section we will illustrate that learning can occur within most participatory action research groups. We have selected to share involved research with people who live with a disabling mental illness.

Background

The motivation for this inquiry was to respond to the concerns of experienced community health workers who worked with people who had mental illness and resided in privately operated supported residential facilities (SRFs) in South Australia (Koch & Kralik, 2002). Community health workers identified that management of urinary and faecal incontinence was having a profound impact on the quality of life for this group of people. For some, incontinence had led to periods of homelessness, for others there were stories of repercussions and out-casting. Incontinence for people living in the community with mental illness was an important health issue that had not previously been addressed.

It is recognized that a significant obstacle in the lives of people living in the community with mental illness is obtaining affordable and secure accommodation:

'Access to appropriate accommodation is regarded by many as the most important determinant in the success or failure of people with chronic mental illness living in the community.'

(Burdekin, 1993, p. 337)

The policy of de-institutionalization for people with mental illness has assumed that people will have somewhere suitable to live in the community with an appropriate level of support. These assumptions have resulted in people with mental illness relying on low-cost accommodation in SRFs. The reality is that SRF accommodation can be substandard or inappropriate for people with mental illness, with little or no opportunity for privacy, occupational therapy or co-ordinated activity. This was a challenging environment in which to seek change.

The research question was: What is the nature and extent of continence problems of residents with mental health conditions living in supported residential facilities, and what can be done to facilitate improvement in their continence status?

The overall aim of this project was to develop continence promotion strategies for people living with mental illness in supported residential facilities. The objectives were to:

(1) develop a participatory, collaborative and transferable model of care that will promote effective management of urinary and faecal incontinence for people living in the community with mental illness;

(2)   identify how key community services can collaborate in order to reduce the incidence of incontinence for people living with mental illness; and

(3)   develop and evaluate training packages and resource materials and disseminate them to services and accommodation providers across Australia, so that they will provide a focus for the management of incontinence for people living with mental illness.

The methodology was guided by participatory action principles. To achieve the aims, the researchers collaborated with three groups: mental health workers, supported residential facility managers, and most importantly, the people residing in the SRFs. A project plan was developed that detailed stages of the project and offered guidance to the project team members, with a view to working towards the project aims and objectives. Ethics approval was obtained from three institutions.

Data were generated from multiple sources. All participants ($n = 37$) were involved in a complete continence assessment and were then guided by the continence advisor for 10 months. This created 117 pages of journal data. Quality of life was measured utilizing the Client Generated Index QOL tool on two occasions at 6-month intervals. The intention was to identify if people participating in the project perceived there had been a shift in their quality of life as a consequence of continence-promoting initiatives and actions.

We facilitated 10 participatory action research group meetings. In separate gender groups, 12 men and 10 women met with us for a total of 10 hours (four participatory action research groups and a follow-up group meeting 4 months later). Individual interviews were also undertaken to explore with people what it was like living with schizophrenia and the effects of antipsychotic medications.

The objective to collaborate with mental health workers and SRF managers was achieved through the implementation of five participatory action group meetings. Data from these meetings were analysed and incorporated to give a comprehensive overview of the political, economic and social contexts that constrain the lives of people with mental illness.

A profile of SRFs in the western Adelaide suburbs (south Australia) was provided. A total of 18 SRFs agreed to participate in this project. A socio-economic analysis was also completed of the history and context of SRFs. A survey of the incidence of resident incontinence in SRFs indicated that 451 or 75% of residents had been diagnosed with a mental illness (including dementia) and 30% were experiencing incontinence. Excluding residents with dementia from these calculations reveals that at least 21% of residents of profiled SRFs diagnosed with a mental illness were reported to also experience problematic incontinence (as reported by managers of SRFs).

All the participants in this study had a debilitating and enduring mental illness. Most participants had been diagnosed with schizophrenia (21 men and 9 women). Schizophrenia is a mental illness characterized by disturbances of thought, perception and a blunting of affect (Coffey, 1998). The illness is associated with a wide range of symptoms that can be inclusive of social withdrawal and disorganized thinking. Many participants experienced short concentration spans, disordered thinking and auditory hallucinations and were socially and economically disadvantaged as a consequence of mental illness (Koch & Kralik, 2002). Participants in this research reported feeling blamed for incontinence because it was perceived by others to be associated with laziness. One participant confided: 'I got kicked out because I wet the bed too much. I was wasting their money'. Incontinence was one reason that residents were evicted from SRFs and as a consequence some participants had endured periods of homelessness.

Nocturnal incontinence was common for these people, and seemed to be often related to the sedative effects of antipsychotic drugs. In close collaboration with participants, individual care plans were developed and responses to the plan discussed, reviewed and modified. People with nocturnal incontinence often felt that they were able to self-manage this problem, but that their mental illness sometimes impacted upon their motivation or often they were too sedated at night to wake. Faecal incontinence was an issue for nine participants, and they tended to be dependent on others to assist with management.

Participatory action research groups

A participatory action research group with 12 men and a group with 12 women were held. Five meetings were held with both groups of people. Then, after a period of 4 months, the groups reconvened for a sixth meeting to determine the sustainability of continence management plans. Other health issues such as diabetes were common (nine participants or 24%) and men talked about the perceived impact of antipsychotic drugs on their sexual lives. Despite the disabling mental health conditions, other health problems and their impoverished social environments, it was noted that the continence status of participants and their quality of life (measured by the CGI) had improved during the research.

SRF residents were provided with shelter, food and assistance with medications; otherwise they were expected to self-care. SRFs are excluded from major government funding programmes and are expected, as private enterprises, to operate for profit. As a consequence, SRF proprietors claim they are unable to offer support to residents that extends beyond the most basic of services to meet minimal human requirements. Hence, continence management and promotion for residents presented a significant challenge in the SRF environment. Incontinence is under-reported in the population of people residing in SRFs because of fear of repercussions. Where possible, residents would try to hide that they had been incontinent. Strategies included hiding soiled linen, cutting holes in mattresses to enable the urine to soak through quicker, wearing multiple layers of clothes and hiding wet clothes. People that live with a mental illness require assistance in managing not only their incontinence but also other health issues.

Using a collaborative research process, participants were facilitated to 'look, think and act'. Avoiding the rhetoric of progress in rehabilitation (Holstein & Gubrium, 2000), where rehabilitation is often described as learning, success was not only the accomplishment of continence but also the way these people were able to incorporate the process of look, think and act into their everyday lives. Separate gender groups were convened because the research team's previous experience was that the separation of gender would permit talk about incontinence that may not otherwise occur. In addition to urinary incontinence, participants placed on the agenda issues such as constipation, faecal incontinence, bed-wetting, impotence and masturbation.

The group meetings were held at a local community centre and lunch and small honorariums were provided to participants in appreciation for their time. The attendance at meetings was relatively stable because the groups were viewed favourably by participants as an opportunity for socialization. We began to notice that some participants attended to their grooming and hygiene on the days that we met.

Researchers facilitated the dynamics of the group, which included: facilitating cross-cultural sensitivities, promoting feelings of equality for all people involved; maintaining harmony; avoiding conflicts; resolving conflicts that arise; encouraging personal, cooperative relationships rather than impersonal, competitive, conflictual or authoritarian relationships; and being sensitive to people's feelings. These sensitivities were discussed at the commencement of the first group with participants, and were identified as 'group norms'. It was necessary to revise the group norms at almost every meeting.

Communication with participants and learning were achieved using diverse approaches. Examples were:

- one to one contact with the continence nurse advisor;
- development of personal care plans;
- guidance and reminders during the course of the project;
- informal educational sessions at participatory action research groups;
- learning from each other in the participatory action research groups;

- multidisciplinary approaches (other health professionals were made aware of the issues and were able to offer reminders); and
- working with managers of SRFs.

It became evident, however, that learning was interrupted during exacerbation of mental illness, but self-care would often recommence following an acute episode.

In the following section we share our reflections of collaboratively researching with people who have debilitating and enduring mental illness. In the spirit of collaboration and participation, we as researchers learnt alongside participants. Whilst we were researching we also asked questions about the participants' experiences of learning to incorporate continence promotion strategies into their lives. To facilitate this mutual learning experience, we asked ourselves: How has the participatory action research process facilitated learning? What were the conditions for learning?

Data analysis techniques used for the participatory action research group data had been previously used and tested and these are presented in Chapter 4. A research coordinator attended and typed verbatim the group dialogue, producing a word-processed record from each meeting on the same day. Data were analysed concurrent to the group meetings. Themes, issues and concerns were extracted and discussed by the research team prior to the next participatory action research meeting. At the subsequent participatory action research meetings, the themes, issues and concerns raised were discussed with the entire group. Each participatory action research group meeting commenced with discussion of the main themes from the previous week, thus this continuous feedback validated the emerging themes. Distinctive features and common themes from each meeting and each group were preserved. The processes of participatory action research, namely 'look, think and act' were clearly evident in these groups and were illustrated by the following examples.

Looking

Together with participants we looked at their lives with incontinence and began to explore what actions they could take that would be suitable for them and the environment in which they lived. A focus on incontinence was being stimulated within the group. Larry shared:

> 'I hate it you know. I'm asleep and I wake up about 4 a.m., the bed is soaking wet and I have to wait till morning. It makes me feel embarrassed, makes me feel unclean. No problems during the day, just at night when I'm asleep. It's only been like that since I've been on Clozapine. I never used to wet the bed . . . Now I am wet every night. I've told the Doctor. I said "Do something for me".'

Until Larry joined the participatory action research group he had been silent about his experiences of bed-wetting. Now that bed-wetting had been discussed in the open, others in the group shared similar stories.

Peter looked at his experiences with incontinence and explored the possibility of the urodome drainage system as potentially making a difference for him. We listened as Jack also considered his experiences with bed-wetting and began to understand that it was occurring at around the same time each night.

Thinking

The story of bed-wetting was common, with nocturnal incontinence being an issue for 18 (48%) of the participants. Participants were convinced that there existed a relationship between antipsychotic medications and nocturnal incontinence. Antipsychotic medications were identified as a major saviour and a culprit. As a saviour, the medication enabled participants to live outside the confines of a mental institution. As a culprit, antipsychotic medications induced a deep sleep that made participants oblivious to the need to urinate or impeded their ability to locate the toilet on time. The sedative effects of antipsychotic drugs taken in the evening sent participants into a heavily sedated state during the night and consequently reduced awareness of bladder sensations, which led to urge incontinence when they woke. Garry thought about his own experiences with nocturnal incontinence:

'I'm on Clozapine – it makes me too relaxed and I don't know what I'm doing. I wake up but too relaxed on these tablets. I'm really tired and I can't get out of bed. Three weeks ago I was in bed sleeping and at 3 a.m. in the morning I feel myself wet, waking up, got into the passageway, don't know where I'm going, so just do it anywhere and go back to bed. The tablets knock you around too much. So you don't know where you're going so you wet yourself, go back to bed. . . . Um, I just don't want to stay in bed with wet blankets over me, it's uncomfortable. I wasn't having the problem before. It's the tablets – Clozapine. The Doctor said you might wet the bed, get fat, I don't care about getting fat. The worse bit is everyone else knows I've wet the bed.'

Thinking was evident when Larry came to the realization that he had a solution for bedwetting and incontinence that came from listening to the experiences of others. Jerry had been thinking about the role his medications were playing in his life. The men in the group had decided they wanted to further understand the effect medications were having on their lives. We invited a community psychiatrist (the prescriber of the medications) to join one meeting and the men asked questions about their medications and discussed the impact of incontinence and impotence on their lives. Although the medication and dosages were often not changed, mutual learning and understanding occurred as explanations were provided and men were included in the decisions of which medications they were prescribed.

Jerry perceived that the early evening sedation was causing long and heavy sleep and consequently he woke with urge incontinence or in a wet bed. When thinking about this, he considered that a container placed close by his bed might be a solution. Here we show that learning occurs as part of interaction with others in the group.

Acting

Acting became evident when Larry was reflecting on his experiences with incontinence and came to the realization that if he 'took half a tablet about 7 p.m. then the others just before bed (he) didn't wet the bed' so he would try dividing his tablets.

'It has worked three or four times for me. I haven't wet the bed. I'm staying up late so don't want to be too sleepy so after the movie is finished I take the rest, don't wet the bed. I take enough to relax me around 7 or 8 p.m. then when tired I pop the rest.'

Larry said that he had 'fluked' this action because it had come about when he had once 'lost half (his) tablets', only to find them and take them later during the evening. The next morning he had woken in a dry bed.

Garry revealed continence promotion strategies that were working for him:

'What I've been doing recently is having a milo at night, get up and go to the toilet, then take my tablets. I don't have any drinks at night-time, if I do I wait and go to the toilet. If I go out I go to the toilet before I go. Things are better now.'

Jerry passed a large volume of urine overnight, and often woke with overwhelming urge incontinence and so found that a continence promotion strategy that worked for him was to keep a bucket by his bed so that he could urinate into it as soon as he woke.

Susan followed the suggestion from other participants to reduce her fluid intake after the evening meal, whilst some participants decided to make it a part of their evening routine to go to the toilet before they went to bed.

Asking questions that stimulated thought and encouraged participants to have a voice facilitated the process of look, think and act. The value of a participatory action research approach was that people were involved in the creation and application of knowledge about them and their worlds based on their own sense making (Reason, 2001). Given that some mental illnesses are accompanied by disordered thinking, it was evident during the meetings that thoughtful responses were stimulated and some participants were immersed in a critically reflective process.

The observation that learning occurs during this participatory action process has been demonstrated. This is not to deny that other ways of working with people, such as one to one exchanges, were not successful. Rather, recognizing that there are others dealing with similar issues and the experience of sharing their stories in the group made the learning process meaningful. We contend that subsequent actions are more likely to be sustained when actions are imbued with meaning and relevant to the context of people's lives.

Towards the completion of the project, most participants perceived that their continence status had improved and they offered some useful suggestions about the participatory action research process. Some men suggested that the meetings 'went too long and we need more smoke breaks' and that 'it takes a while to finish conversations . . . listening to everyone in the group'. Others suggested that 'it was good to learn new things, such as using an extra bottle (urinal) at night'. The participants were pleased to learn that there had been a national outcome from their involvement: 'It's good that a book is being compiled'. For others, it was important that they had been heard: 'I discussed bed wetting for the first time'. Women found benefit in the interaction with others: 'I like coming here, I learnt about myself and the (pelvic floor exercises)'. They also enjoyed learning and sharing continence promotion strategies that may have relevance for them: 'It is an outing . . . I like being with people and I learned about exercises, kylie sheets and buckets'.

The argument advanced here is that provision of education is not always enough to ensure changes in self-care, but what could be offered to compliment health education programmes is a process similar to the participatory action research approach described here. Research has revealed that individuals need to understand how to use new information, and to learn ways in which they can incorporate it into their lives (Kralik et al., 2004). Self-care occurs when the person is able to establish a sense of order in daily life. It is a process in which the individual perceives, manages and takes action in response to the symptoms and disability that the disease presents. During this inquiry, participants identified strategies for continence promotion that were relevant and possible for their own lives. They were not forced to adopt strategies that were beyond their capacity or did not fit with their lives or the environment in which they lived. People were facilitated towards constructing continence self-care strategies by using their own knowledge and experiences because people 'are to some significant degree self-determining . . . that is to say that they are the authors of their own actions' (Reason, 1994, p. 325). Using the 'look, think and act' process encouraged participants to reflect on their situation and to establish a plan for action.

What are the conditions under which understanding and learning were made possible?

The interactions between facilitator and participants are closely observed and recorded during participatory action research group meetings. When 12 people participate in a group discussion, the facilitator remains alert. Jimmy is a young man living with a disabling mental health condition and urinary incontinence. The second author, while facilitating a participatory action research group, recorded the following observations:

> 'Jimmy is agitated, sitting forward in his chair and rocking. I can feel him staring at me. I can tell he wants to go outside to have a smoke. People are talking, sharing and reflecting on their experiences of wetting the bed, so I don't want the group to break just yet. I look at Jimmy and smile; he returns the smile and makes a gesture as if he is zipping his lips closed. We understand each other. He sits back in his chair and nods at me. I ask the men: "What information has been useful for you?" Colin says: "I'm still trying to go to the loo whenever I can, once after and before a meal. Cutting down on fluids, only have about three drinks instead of five. Cross my fingers I hope to be dry tonight." Jon says: "The awareness factor – over the last 3 weeks we have been taught to be more aware of our waterworks. Can't ignore the fact that I'm going to need to go to the loo during the night, so I make sure that the urinal is empty. If I take my medication later at night I know I can get a good night's sleep."'

Creating an environment and opportunities conducive for learning is central to the participatory action research process. Participants were together over an extended period of time so they developed friendships and support networks. As they became more comfortable with one another they felt safe to express what they were thinking and feeling without fear of judgement. The perception of safety was critical for meaningful communication to occur. Group members provided each other with social and emotional support. Group norms were expressed and self-monitored. Jimmy knew when to zip his lips.

Recognition is given to the diversity of perspectives that a participatory action research group assembles. An environment conducive to learning opens the door to the variety of views but at the same time engages individuals in identifying self-care strategies that have meaning in their lives. It is critical that the group engage extensively in listening to one another's stories and being open to how each individual attaches meaning to the illness experience. Sharing experiences was usual, yet what individuals take on board from the exchange is not a rigidly prescribed formula for coping with their chronic illness. Participants take on board information or another's experience when it has meaning or relevance in their situation. They assume the right to construct their own story of life with illness.

'Look, think and act' cycles are instigators of dialogue and action, as 'true reflection leads to action' (Freire, 1970, p. 41). Through story telling, participatory action research encourages participants to explore their own experiences. Reflection often initiates transition or moving on towards incorporating a chronic condition into one's life. A participatory action research approach carries a fundamental rhythm of learning through reflection and action, during which participants open themselves to more subtle understandings and engagement with the process. Taking control gave satisfaction to participants and was evidenced in the way they were empowered to incorporate self-care strategies into their lives, creating a sense of accomplishment. Our experiences with people who participated in this research inquiry have confirmed that people with schizophrenia respond positively to this approach to care. Health workers practising participatory caring have a heightened sense of engagement in contrast to a practise of avoidance, distancing and ultimately detachment (Kralik et al., 1997).

Most important was the facilitation of critical reflection within the group so that participants did not feel blamed for incontinence, but could view it as an issue requiring action and resolution. Collaboration and prolonged engagement with SRF managers and staff meant that empathy and understanding often replaced the blame environment. Wetting the bed was no longer perceived to be a behavioural issue. In these changed environments, many participants began to trust themselves to direct their own self-care strategies.

Openness to other interpretations was important, as participants discovered that hearing the experiences of others helped them to learn. When participants shared their experiences they permitted other views to be considered and to be entwined with their own understandings. Participants experienced a growth in self-knowledge because they were provided with the opportunity to be central to decision making, judging the self-care strategies and decisions on the basis of their appropriateness, personal meaningfulness and significance (Paterson et al., 2002; Kralik et al., 2004).

Awareness of self can be advanced, which will 'free them to be more than passive objects' (Freire, 1970, p. 23). Rather than offer participants a structured education programme, we suggest that the participatory action research process facilitated reflection and learning. A focus was provided on what was possible for individuals and the environment in which they lived. Primacy was placed on practical knowing. The participatory action research process was empowering because the focus was to identify the potential for development rather than the deficits of participants.

Thoughtfulness acknowledges the need to incorporate the views of clients in care (Northway, 2000). There exists a risk that researchers will merely pay lip service to such an approach or that it will be conducted in a 'top down' manner (Northway, 2000). This has often been the case with client groups that have been perceived to be difficult to consult, such as people with debilitating and enduring mental illness.

Willingness for all participants to try to understand 'the others' is a condition for learning. It is not possible for some people to be open (either through choice or capability), but we foster an awareness that as participants we bring our own experiences, values and interests to each situation. It is acknowledged throughout the participatory action research process that divergent views are expressed from different backgrounds, experience and knowledge bases and that this may open participants' minds to new ways of thinking. Listening to different ways of looking at the world is possibly a condition for learning to take place.

George's story

The opportunity for context to be understood from one to one interviews needs to be acknowledged. Here we share a conversation with George, who was a 42-year-old physically large man. We suspect he paid particular attention to his hygiene and dress on the days that he met with us because he perceived participation in the project as an 'outing'. He had a sharp wit and an engaging sense of humour. Diabetes aside, his protruding 'belly' was testament to a fondness for food. We listened as George talked about his life with schizophrenia, living in a boarding house and the challenges confronting him.

Being diagnosed

George described the protracted and difficult period in his life before he received a medical diagnosis and psychiatric treatment:

'When I was nineteen I was told to see a psychiatrist but I didn't till I was 25. I got sick in 1985. I remember that I would hibernate in my room. My sister would come over and tell me to get out of bed and have a shower. I wouldn't shower for months. Then one day I drove to my sister's place – I left my car in the middle of the road. I didn't know what was going on. I started screaming out. I was having a nervous breakdown. The coppers came and put me in the back seat. They said take him to Hillcrest. I ran for my life. But they caught me. They took me to Hillcrest. I went off me tree. Mum and Dad came and saw me. They were shocked, I was really round the bend. All these voices in my head. I didn't have a job because I wasn't well. I didn't get a pension. I kept saying I'd get well. That's why I'm still here on the planet.'

George has moved on from his time of diagnosis. He is reconciled to his illness and perceives his approach and responses to the impact of schizophrenia to be different from those of other people he has known:

'Yes, I am diagnosed with schizophrenia. I'm not the only one though. Years ago people would just give up. But I'm not like that. Most of my good friends are dead. One of my friends hanged himself at his farm. Another woman died in hospital.'

The early experiences of living with schizophrenia were not unlike those of others who came to a slow realization that something was wrong with their mental health. People around them often observed bizarre behaviours but it was not until a crisis occurred that intervention for treatment was possible.

Medication: the saviour and the culprit

Medication was central to his life. George identified an antipsychotic medication called Clozapine, in particular, as both a major saviour and culprit affecting his life. Sleeping in a semicomatose state 12 hours a day was typical, and drowsiness in his waking hours was evident. The many side-effects made life more complex and difficult but George knew that he needed the medication in order to function in the community:

'The psychiatrist and I talked for a long time before I went on Clozapine because it can kill you. I had to sign a bit of paper. Suddenly I was on it. It's a good drug but half my days are gone because I can't get up and I can't eat properly. Since Clozapine I've been all right. With my mental illness I have it under control. I am doing all right. I'm all right now as long as I keep well. But I go to hospital for a rest every 2 or 3 years.'

'I'm well as long as I keep taking tablets. I do get stressed at night-time. I don't know why. I thought I wanted to talk to someone about what is on my mind. I get depressed at night-time. I've got to that stage again. I'm not sick, I don't hear voices. I'm a bit stressed lately. If I move out I'll get the same situation or whatever. I don't know where to go for help. I can't sort out what to do with my life. I can't really go back to work, that's the killer bit. If I go over the border I have to get my tablets you see. That's why I buy x-lotto. I think about pissing off. The main thing I do is take my tablet. I haven't eaten today because I can't get up in time.'

Not worrying about diabetes

The complexities of life with schizophrenia were compounded by diabetes; however, he chose to ignore this condition. He knew what he should do to gain control of his high blood glucose levels but was unable to transfer that knowledge into his everyday living:

'Um, I don't know. I don't think there is nothing wrong. I don't worry about it. I don't know what's happening.'

Coping with daily life amidst schizophrenia was all consuming, and there was little capacity to also deal with the restrictions of a diabetes diet.

Feeling trapped

George revealed an overwhelming sense of being trapped in his current situation of poverty, social isolation and boredom. Mundane outings for blood tests and collection of medications provided a distraction in the day:

'I'm sick of lining up for a meal and stuff like that. I'd like a little extra money. I'd like to manage my money and cigarettes. I don't want to stay there and put up with TV. That's not life for me . . . there's more out there. There is no point sitting around and watching TV. I go and have a blood test. That gets me out for a while. That's an outing. Picking up tablets on Tuesday is an outing. I'm trapped. I'm only getting $10 a week for dishes. I can't get a full-time job because they put it in public trustee and I'm working for nothing. You think to yourself your life has finished. You gotta keep going but I have given up a lot.'

George wanted more for his life, but this seemed beyond his grasp. A personal vision for the future was obstructed and possibilities for taking action in the areas of his life that were important for him were denied.

Feeling abandoned

A sense of abandonment from significant others in his life was profound. Mental illness imposed on the possibility of forming close relationships, which created dark voids of loneliness and boredom in his days. He was drawn to the childhood memories of security and nurturing from his parents, but was aware that they found it difficult to 'handle' him:

'Not many people go to their family for lunch because they don't want them, even some of my family don't want me. Mum said last year she can't handle me, so I think about that all the time. All these memories! I couldn't keep it to myself. I go to Mum's but I get depressed when I go back (to the SRF). I went to see Mum because it's normal and that's what I feel in my heart. When I go home I get depressed again.'

Deciding what is important

The restrictions on George's life were keenly felt. He had little choice in how daily life was constructed or little direction for his future. Travelling was important, but paying for rent and food at the SRF used up most of his government sourced income. What little money was left over was spent on cigarettes, coffee and 'hot chips'. He turned his focus towards winning money and sometimes thought of stealing so he could achieve his dreams. Money was perceived as empowering and the key to a changed life with a secure future:

'I want to keep well and get some money to get going. All I need is to win $25,000, give Mum and Dad $1000 each, have a party and get on a bus to WA, train ride on the Ghan. I don't want to sit around and watch the TV. Travelling is fun. I want to change my life. Yes I want to change my life. Sometimes in my head because I want money I feel like breaking in and taking someone's money. I don't want to sit here and keep on saying it. I want to get a life – you can't get one in a boarding house. It's different if you're sick. I feel that if I'm well I should do what I want to do. I've told that story lots of times. That's life. I can't stay home and watch TV all my life, can I? Shit what a life, hey? What a situation! What am I going to do? Sit around, drink coffee and watch the idiot box? Well I just want my money to go away. This is why people commit suicide because they can't do what they want to do.'

George's story revealed that the symptoms of schizophrenia shaped every aspect of his life and intruded upon any sense of certainty for the future. Clozapine, in particular, was identified as having a major impact on daily life. The medication, however, meant George was able to live outside the confines of a mental health institution.

Access and equity: the implications for health practice

Although the focus has been on the experience of living with schizophrenia, health professionals care for many people in the community with mental illness. There is bountiful evidence that these people are often disadvantaged in both the acute and community health care sectors. People with mental illness require access to a full range of treatment and rehabilitation services to lessen the impairment and disruption produced by their condition. In terms of equity, we should offer people living in boarding type housing, assistance in navigating access to available community health services. This project has provided some new understandings about the experience of having a mental illness that should challenge the practice of health professionals. Driven by primary health care principles, community health workers can play an important part in the development of comprehensive care for this client group. It is paramount for community care that has meaning in the lives of people, that health workers acknowledge the challenges confronting people with mental illness, and provide care within a holistic framework that incorporates the clients' social, physical, spiritual and emotional needs.

In this chapter we have provided details from two inquiries to demonstrate the way in which learning can and does take place in a supported environment. We have demonstrated that the participatory action research process facilitates understanding and meaning. These people had been able to incorporate the process of look, think and act into their everyday lives. However, the claim that the look, think and act process continues to resonate in participants' lives once researchers have left the field has yet to be evaluated.

6 Preparation of Community Practitioners in Everyday Practice

What is the difference between participatory action and participatory action research?

Participatory action without research is a useful process in everyday health care practice. The participatory action process involves working with people towards self-devised plans and sustained outcomes. It is not unlike the nursing process of assess, plan, implement and evaluate, except participation with client/community is privileged. Participatory action leaves behind the problem focus and prescriptive standardized care plans of the nursing process. Rather, participatory action focuses on capacity building and/or identifying people's strengths. Participatory action processes instigate and promote collaboration with clients/community, leaving behind professional dictates. The resultant mutually agreed health care plan or agenda for action relies on matters raised by the people themselves. The role of the health care professional is to walk alongside the client/community as an active participant in health promotion or in some situations towards death. Precisely because we are building capacity, the process is likely to be sustained once the collaborative relationship between the health care professional and the client and/or community has ended. By capacity building we refer to those activities and actions that give an individual, community and/or population sustained ability for growth, development or accomplishment.

Investment and ownership of the agenda by clients/community secures sustainability of the action plan and its outcomes. Plans and outcomes are recorded, monitored and stored for retrieval for legal and quality reasons. Health promotion and educational preparation of health care practitioners as participants rather than experts needs to be formalized. Participatory action leads the client towards choice and control.

In this chapter we argue that participatory action can encourage health care practitioners to work alongside their clients and community. Primary health care principles inform this approach. Since the 1970s the meaning of health promotion has shifted from an emphasis on instructing individuals to take up healthy behaviours to recognizing that their social environment shapes people's actions. The Ottawa Charter illustrates this shift and goes beyond earlier individual and behavioural definitions. This social health agenda assumes that inequalities in health care can be examined and changed through the manipulation of socio-economic or structural health determinants (gender, age, class or ethnicity). This movement constitutes the New Public Health approach to health promotion and seeks to advance the interests of groups disadvantaged by gender, age, class or ethnicity. It requires a shift in thinking about health promotion, from it being related to lifestyle behaviours, prevention of disease and disability, to include wider social and political reform. The challenge to promote health between sectors (e.g. human services, transport and health) requires collaboration between governments, health and other economic sectors. One other important justification for us to use a participatory action approach is that the principles are closely aligned to the primary health care concepts of collaboration and empowerment. Primary health care emphasizes the participation of people in the planning and development of their own health care, and this is an important foundation for our evidence-based community nursing practice.

Primary health care principles

Ideally, health care is organized within an integrated team and supported by a community network that includes as partners not only the health care workers and service providers but also the community itself. In addition, an approach to health care based on primary health care principles is valid for both acute and community care settings.

A primary health care approach moves beyond the individual and the medical and/or nursing diagnosis (clinical and curative approach) to view the larger social picture of people in the context of socio-economic, cultural and political environment. The primary health care approach considers the way in which the context affects health and then acts upon this information. The principles of primary health care give attention to social justice, equity, community participation and responsiveness to needs. We can acknowledge that one's health status may be related to poverty and socioeconomic status. We know that poverty, dirty water and tobacco often means early death. We know that communities are strengthened by social cohesion. We can also see the impact of inequality when health care is not affordable or when access to health services is denied. Encouraging or facilitating health practice with people requires first that we consider what we mean by the term 'health'. Our interpretation is that individual health is a state of physical, mental and social well-being and not merely the absence of disease or infirmity. Wass (2001) widens the perspective to say that:

'The health of individuals is strongly influenced by the social, cultural, political and economic conditions of the society in which they live and it can never be fully considered outside that context.'

(Wass, 2001, p. 45)

As health care professionals we can take into account the principle of social justice but we may feel that the agenda for change and reform is beyond the scope of our everyday practice. We are concerned about equity and we strive, on behalf of clients and the community, for accessible and responsive health services. The role of health care professionals in implementing the principles of primary health care is central to the concept of 'health for all'. Health care professionals are challenged to embrace a leadership role in the promotion of primary health care. Here we discuss ways that primary health care principles of participation and responsiveness can become central to practice.

Participation

In this section we emphasize the primary health care principles of participation and responsiveness to needs. Working *with* clients and communities is the most appropriate primary health care strategy for health care professionals. Participation has been described as the heart of primary health care (Wass, 2001) and assumes that members of the community have expertise regarding their own lives and the issues that affect them. The role of health workers is to have knowledge and expertise of their particular field rather than assuming expertise in aspects of people's lives. Simply put, the health worker may be the expert in clinical matters, but the client is the expert in his or her own life. Indeed, thinking about new ways to work with individual clients (and relevant stakeholders) is the challenge. Here we consider a health practice focus that provides people with the means to grow and learn in a participative relationship. Whilst our research focus has been chronic illness, we suggest that many of the principles are transferable to all areas of health care.

Working with people

Our health care systems are not always designed with the client in mind and often do little to assist clients to care for themselves. Instead, our health care is based on an old acute-care model, where the nurse tells the client what to do to get better. The client's role is often passive.

That model does not work well for people learning to live the rest of their lives with chronic illness. The health care professional is still very much the authority, trying to get the client to do what is needed; the client's job is simply to be obedient. What we've found, however, is that you can't get people to 'do' anything. The motivation to change one's behaviour, even to take one's medication, comes largely from within us. The client is responsible and must be central to his or her own care.

Some questions raised may be: Why can't we stay with the old health care models? Why does the client need to be so involved? We suggest there are several reasons. First, most chronic illness care does not even involve nurses and other health care professionals. Instead, most health care is given by the person who has the illness. On a day-to-day basis, the client is in charge of his or her own health, and the daily decisions people make have a huge impact on client outcomes and quality of life.

Assessment is the cornerstone of health care practice, essentially occurring at two levels: the individual and the community/population. We talk about primary health care principles but what do they really mean in the scope of our everyday practice? According to the traditional biomedical model, professionals are the ultimate decision-makers. Inclusion of clients in decision-making is often given perfunctory status. The failure of the traditional models of care for some people has led us to ask: What kind of approach can we use to work with people? In other words, how can we change health care practice so that it has meaning for people and better fits with their experiences? Many research participants have expressed the need for health workers to change their approach to practice:

> 'It's just struck me how authoritative and knowledgeable many of the suggestions have been and that this is interesting in informing the basis of our group. If our medical practitioners could just see us as the group of capable women we are, rather than as a set of medical "problems" I feel everyone's life would be much easier.'

Listening as an assessment strategy

Guided by primary health care principles, there is potential in the nursing process for listening to clients to occur. Using listening as an assessment strategy depends on the individual nurse and his/her understanding of the significance of working *with* clients in establishing mutually agreed-upon goals for care. It is important that we find out from people what have been their experiences of our nursing so that we can make creative changes to our practice.

Box 6.1   Participatory learning and action in nursing (PLAN).

PLAN   Reflective practice questions that can be applied to
                your reading, events in your practice and/or your life.

LOOK   • Describing
                  — What is happening here?

THINK   • Informing
                  — What does this mean?
                  — How did I come to be like this? Why do I think
                    this way?
                • Deconstructing and/or confronting
                  — Do I need to challenge certain taken-for-
                    granted assumptions that are evident in
                    my thinking/practice/life?
                  — What can I do to move on?

ACT   • Reconstructing
                  — How might I do things differently?
                • Evaluate
                  — How will I know things have changed?

Maintaining a daily journal offers a strategy that can help clinicians address some troublesome practice-based issues and reflect on practice. Telling stories about your work makes practice visible. What nurses do in one day is much more than the organizational statistics that currently measure practice. Perhaps we should take the initiative and describe practice as we view it. Stories generated from practice have the potential to bring nursing practice and subsequent action into harmony. Here it is suggested that journal keeping is a pivotal activity in clinical practice. However, this process requires analytical skills to move it beyond mere documentation. Writing, analysing, reflecting and rewriting are skills that do not come easily to some practitioners. The 'look, think and act' process used to guide participatory action research can also be used in participatory action and offers a legitimate practice approach for the health professional (Box 6.1).

Is primary health care time consuming?

It is often said that health care professionals do not have time to embrace primary health care principles. The four principles of primary health care are equity, social justice, health promotion and working *with* clients and communities. One of the best ways to work *with* a community is in responsiveness to its needs. In this section we explore how to assess the needs of a group so that we can respond.

Participatory action and feminist approaches in research have gained attention during the last few years. Both approaches are participative and collaborative and congruent with primary health care principles. In this book we have emphasized primary health care principles: social justice, equity, responsiveness to needs and participation. You may ask what has a research strategy to do with the participatory approach you may use when working with groups or individuals? We suggest that the principles are similar and may be adapted for use in everyday practice. Again we talk about the participatory action process as 'look, think and act' and have signalled that this approach is useful for reflective practice as well as working with clients. In the following section we will draw on recent research that shows the way in which the principles of participatory action research can be practised in the community. It is a possible strategy for working with individual clients and the community, and it may be an appropriate approach to consider when undertaking a community assessment.

Participatory action in practice

Reviewing earlier critical points, the four guiding principles that define participatory action research (Stringer, 1999) are that it is a process that is:

- democratic, enabling participation of all people;
- equitable, acknowledging people's equality of worth;
- liberating, providing freedom from oppressive, debilitating conditions; and
- life enhancing, enabling the expression of people's full human potential.

Participatory action

Community based action research is a collaborative approach to inquiry and provides people with the means to take systematic action to resolve the issues confronting them. As discussed, this approach favours consensual and participatory procedures that enable the participants to set the agenda for discussion, to prioritize issues they wish to discuss, and devise plans to deal with the issues at hand. Taken into account are the participants' accounts of history, culture, interactional practices and emotional lives.

Although we talk about *participatory action research*, health care professionals can use *participation* and *action* in everyday practice without the research element. Hence we use the term 'participatory action'. The look, think and act process can be very useful in everyday practice. We repeat: *Looking* means gathering information, and defining and describing the situation. *Thinking* refers to exploring, analysing, interpreting and explaining. Thinking is stimulated as participants ask 'What is happening here?' and 'Why are things as they are?'. *Acting* refers to the development of plans devised by participants, followed by implementation and evaluation.

Applying these principles, participatory action enables participants to systematically investigate their issues, formulate experiential accounts and then devise plans to deal with them. Cycles of collaborative issue identification, planning, action and evaluation are repeated in a series of iterations so that improved understanding of the nature of the issues and effective solutions are developed. Participatory action is useful for issues that are not well understood because they are complex and multi-dimensional. This is particularly the case in cross-cultural situations where the issue of health programme responsiveness requires the inclusion of all stakeholders in the exploration of programme changes. Without the participation of all those involved, commitments to proposed changes are unlikely. The participatory action process can lead to theoretical development and action can take place at individual or collective levels. A participant may plan to try alternative ways of managing his/her condition, or the participatory action group may agree on a larger reform strategy, such as lobbying for improved health services.

Participatory action aims to demonstrate a culturally sensitive way of working with people and seeks to change the social and personal dynamics of the research situation. The approach is non-competitive, non-exploitative, seeks to enhance the lives of those who participate, and assumes cooperation and consensus are a primary focus of research. Stringer (1999, p. 21) argues that participatory action seeks 'viable, sustainable, and effective solutions to common issues through dialogue and negotiation'.

Participatory action and client education

Just as client-centred care can be more effective, client-centred education is more effective education. The older style education programme, where we sit people down and lecture to them, does not work. Its effectiveness is no better than sitting them down and telling them to 'lose 20 kilos' or 'stop smoking'. There is no acknowledgement of the context of the person's life, their needs or values. The client's needs can effectively drive the education. For example, education can be based entirely on questions from the client. As a clinician with expertise and knowledge, you may have a checklist of topics you want to cover, but those topics can be addressed in the context of client questions rather than through an impersonal lecture. Clients usually are not as interested in the biophysical nature of disease as health workers may be. They want to know the illness or condition in relation to the context of their lives. What does this mean to me? How will this make life different for me?

All of us are engaged in a life-long learning process and central to our role as health workers is to engage with people in order to support learning. Most people that we work with and who have a condition that has brought them into contact with health workers manage themselves for the majority of the time. Health workers simply play a support role. It is important that people know they have options. There is rarely one perfect way to treat a condition. Clients need to understand the different treatment options available and should be encouraged to look at the personal costs and benefits of each.

With support from health workers, people can change their behaviour, but it may take time to do so. Assure them that they will have your support. Rarely do clients leave the doctor's office and immediately enact whatever change was recommended. Life is full of changes and fluctuations. What works one day might not work the next. Talk with clients about significant behavioural changes that can be made by setting goals, taking that first step and figuring out what they may learn about themselves along the way.

Helping clients set self-care goals

The driving force behind each client visit is the client's agenda or goals related to his or her condition. Ideally, the goal is clearly displayed in the client's plan of care, and each person who handles the plan plays a part in supporting the client in that goal, asking: How did it go? What have you done this week? How can we help you do better?

The process of setting 'self-care' goals with the individual client involves essentially three steps.

(1) Look . . . Find the issue. Rather than beginning the client encounter focused on test results, begin by saying, 'Tell me what concerns you most. Tell me what is hardest for you. Tell me what you're most distressed about and what you'd most like to change.'

(2) Think . . . When you begin to get a sense of the client's concerns, explore those issues together. Ask: 'Is there an underlying issue? Do you really want this issue to be solved?'

(3) Act . . . Develop a collaborative goal and action to achieve it. Once you have worked with the client to identify the issue, your instinct may be to try to solve it, but don't. Instead, validate the client's feelings and his or her capacity to deal with the issue, and continue asking questions that will lead the client to his or her own solution. Ask: 'What do you think would work? What have you tried in the past? What would you like to try?'

It is always more meaningful when people find the 'ah ha!' on their own, and it is important to give them that opportunity. Encourage the person to come up with ideas first, then offer your own suggestions or additional information that they may need. You can say 'This works for some people', 'Have you tried this?' or 'Here's why that may not be a great idea'. The important thing is to give the person the opportunity to make the final decision on what goal to try.

At the end of the conversation, the client will be able to tell you one step he or she is going to try. Encourage them to be specific. If the client says, 'I'm going to exercise more', ask what that means. Will they exercise three times a week? What exercise will they do? Help them to come up with a specific plan that they have created for themselves. From a health worker's perspective, what clients envisage for themselves may not be the goal you would have chosen for them, but it is one they see as being possible in their lives, hence they are more likely to accomplish it. Sandra described how she set about making changes following a turbulent time with illness:

'So on a very conscious level I decided to start with something small. Something big seemed too hard to me. So I started with something really tiny, and the rainbows came after the storm. The tiny window of light peaked through and then I was more able to pry the door open so I could see opportunities to make changes in my life.'

During further contact with the person, you can build upon the existing plan, continually looking at the issues, thinking about possibilities and revising the planned actions. As health workers have infrequent contact with people, we usually only see the outer shell of a person; rarely do we even begin to understand or realize their past experiences, hopes, dreams or memories that remain hidden from view, but are central to shaping the way they live their lives.

Who actually works with clients to set and revise their actions and goals on an ongoing basis, whether it is you or another health worker, is less important than the notion that clients are encouraged to be the decision makers. The emphasis on self-care goals suggests that the care is for them. It is their agenda, and they are active participants in the outcome.

Empowering clients with information

Depending on the health setting you are working in, one way to help clients focus and begin thinking about health care goals is to talk with them about their individual health measures (such as blood results, blood pressure, HbA1c) and what those numbers mean. People who we have researched with have shared how important it has been to them when living with a long-term illness to have access to test results. One research participant said:

> 'I find having the results and reports invaluable. I can compare my results with previous ones and know exactly whether or not I'm improving, I'm static or if my levels are dropping.'

Offering explanation of what the numbers mean (ideal and actual) can lead to conversations about strategies for improvement or stabilization. When faced with results from tests, clients may see for themselves where they may be struggling and what they can do to better their results. Andrew sees great benefit in this approach:

> 'I think I have always been a "practical" person but my illness has made me more so. I find that sympathy is much less important to me – either giving or receiving, but rather want to get on with finding a solution. It has made me harder and stronger and probably made me somewhat detached from people emotionally. I still value people, but in a different way.'

> 'Becoming more practical is a bit of a survival skill: living with a chronic illness which requires continual monitoring means I cannot afford to "fall in a heap", somehow I just have to continue to look after myself.'

Health workers often feel most helpful when giving advice. It may be, however, that we rarely help people to address confronting issues or make lasting changes in their lives simply by telling them what they should do. Ultimately, clients need to find their own solutions and motivation and must take responsibility for their health. We can be important cogs in a life-long learning process that can empower clients to do just that.

Health workers can best facilitate people towards self-care by embracing new understandings of the experience of learning to live with long term illness. This process is enhanced when the expertise a person brings to the management of their condition is given the respect it deserves. Consider a practice focus that provides people with the means to grow and learn in a participative relationship.

Box 6.2 Working principles of participatory action.

Principle	Qualities
Relationships that are:	Equal
	Harmonious
	Accepting
	Cooperative
	Sensitive
Communication that is:	Attentive
	Accepting
	Comprehensible
	Truthful
	Sincere
	Appropriate
	Advisory
Participation that is:	Involving
	Active
	Supportive
	Successful
	Personal
Inclusion that accounts for:	All individuals
	All groups
	All issues
	Cooperation
	Benefit

(Stringer, 1999, p. 46, adapted by Susan Mann 2002)

Guiding principles of participatory action

While a participatory action approach to working with people may appear to be fundamental, it is a complex undertaking. Box 6.2 summarizes these working principles.

Participatory action and working with groups of people

Often health practice requires that we work with groups of people. Facilitation skills are paramount when working with community. Group dynamics are expressed in the typical life of a group as forming, storming, norming, performing and mourning (Wass, 2001). There are also suggestions about leadership, power, influence, decision-making and group goals. When working with groups, the following should be considered:

- ideal numbers of people for a group;
- timing of groups (at what time and for how long to meet);
- location for meeting;
- seating arrangements at meetings;
- getting the group 'started'; and
- facilitating group discussion.

Setting the scene: preliminary activity for participatory action groups

In order to create an environment that is supportive and encouraging, the group participants will need to be a part of developing that environment. This is assisted by discussion and agreement on guidelines that will create a culture within the group, which will make it easy for people to discuss their ideas and share their knowledge and experience.

The first meeting

Formulate questions that you think would be useful to ask when you meet with the group:

- Why are we meeting today?
- What is/are the issue/s?
- How does it affect our work/lives?
- Who is being affected?
- What are the things that are happening?
- When are things happening?

Discuss, clarify and agree on questions to be asked of participants in the community group. Items to consider:

- Recruitment of participants
- Deciding on the number of participants
- Setting the scene, the environment, refreshments
- Structuring the first session
- Preparing the agenda
- Resources (literatures, 'experts', access to the web)
- The time frame per session/number of sessions
- Agreeing on group norms

- Issue identification, e.g. Why are you running the group?
- Promoting feelings of equality for all people involved
- Role of the facilitator, e.g. resolving conflicts that arise, managing group dynamics
- Recording and analysis
- Closure (when you cease working with the group)
- Writing the paper/report (with whom?)
- Disseminating the findings (to whom?)
- Other aspects not listed above?

Health promotion

Congruent with a basic tenet of primary health care, health promotion intrinsically involves working *with* people. As also previously discussed, health promotion ideally is more than health education. These ideals are the main focus of this book, especially with regard to promoting health for individuals. Emphasis has moved away from solely educating individuals, towards recognizing the power of education to help create healthy environments. Here it is argued that is not useful to think simplistically that giving a person more information about a health issue will change attitudes and stimulate changes in health behaviours. Here we point to the difference between health education and health promotion. Moving towards a more humanistic and encompassing paradigm (rather than a biomedical paradigm) for providing care and health promotion will assist nurses to promote health more success-fully. Remaining focused on the principles of primary health care and applying these principles to the conduct of education should be the aim. Working *with* participants to establish their needs and working with clients and community to promote health, means thinking about notions of equity, social justice and empowerment. This can be an empowering experience for both the client and the nurse. Therefore, primary health care principles can direct, and be embedded within, the evaluation process.

Evaluation

In nursing contexts, it can be argued that the goals of evaluation research are to provide evidence about our practice, service or pro-grammes. This evidence is deemed necessary for decision making, not only by those who provide the funding for our programmes, but also by us in demonstrating accountability for our work. Evidence procured in this way provides assurances of quality in our practices. Those who fund health services and programmes want to be reassured that health outcomes are achieved and that the interventions we provide make a difference to the lives of clients and the wider community. Indeed, evidence provided by evaluation can be used to convince funding agencies, communities and clients that our services, programmes and projects are necessary and viable. As Wass (2001, p. 124) writes: '... the daily practice of an individual health worker, the overall work of an agency or team, and specific health promotion activities or projects will all benefit from regular evaluation'. Not only should we take charge of our own evaluations, evaluating *with* stakeholders will provide evidence that our programmes, services and practices are relevant for clients and the wider community. The focus will be on taking responsibility for evaluations that affect our lives, our services, our programmes and our professions.

We have argued that our programmes, services and practices are evaluated and that we evaluate collaboratively. The central evaluation question is, 'are people accomplishing what they want to accomplish?' Collaborative evaluation, utilizing the same principles as participatory action research, includes stakeholders in the evaluation (Koch, 2003). Evaluation research includes 'any effort to increase human effectiveness through systematic data based inquiry'. Being *systematic* is the operating word. A central notion driving this type of evaluation is negotiation. Collaborative evaluation:

- involves all participants affected by the evaluation;
- invites participants research alongside the evaluator;
- integrates programme development and implementation from the very beginning;
- incorporates evaluation data throughout the life of a project so that actions become more congruent with evolving goals;
- identifies views that may be in conflict and creates a safe place for their engagement; and
- integrates a new thinking process into an organization's culture.

This then takes us full circle to where we commenced this section of the book, wondering about how best the health needs of an individual can be facilitated, how health can be promoted in the fullest sense (holistically from a more than individualistic perspective) at all levels, how health promotion can be evaluated, and how the principles of primary health care can be effectively pursued throughout.

7 Facilitation

We have shared some of the insights gained while researching with people who live with HIV and fatigue, those who have a disabling mental illness and people who expertly self-manage their asthma. In so doing we may have understated the need for expert facilitation.

Role of the facilitator

Stringer's (1996) guidelines on the role of facilitator are particularly useful. A researcher, within the traditional paradigms, is an 'expert' carrying out research, whereas participatory action research has evolved to a point where the researcher is a 'resource' person and referred to as facilitator, associate or consultant. The participatory action research facilitator acts as a catalyst to assist participants to define their concerns clearly, and then support them as they find solutions. The facilitator can achieve this by using the following guidelines:

- Stimulate, rather than impose change. Encourage participants to change through addressing issues that concern them now.
- Focus on the way things are done, rather than using the traditional method of focusing on results achieved.
- Ensure that the process starts where people are, rather than where someone else thinks they are, or where someone thinks they ought to be.
- Assist participants to analyse their present situation, consider what they find and then plan for what parts they would like to keep and what they would like to change.

However, it is not the role of the facilitator to tell the participants what they should change or keep, but rather to respect and acknowledge the participants' ideas (Stringer, 1999), and enable participants to view several options and consider the potential outcomes or consequences of those options. When the participants have selected an option, it is the facilitator's role to assist with the implementation of the plan by identifying the pros and cons and then helping to locate the necessary resources. It is recognized that the ultimate responsibility for the success of the process centres on the participants. They need a feeling of 'ownership' and thus motivation to invest time and energy in order to change the status quo.

The facilitator leads the group where it wants to go; the outcomes of the participatory action research process cannot be predicted. The facilitator has to learn to live with uncertainties.

Understanding how to live with uncertainties

We are attracted to the notion of human flourishing, particularly when this refers to the clients of health services. We sense a need for participative approaches in health care as its practices have traditionally been controlled by medicine as the dominant paradigm (Kralik et al., 2001b). It is usual for the receiver of health care services to be named the patient. The patient has been defined as an object, to be manipulated by treatments controlled by the medical practitioner. Even now, the current mantra is that people should be given education to become patients and comply with prescriptive self-management regimes. Whilst the rhetoric is self-management of chronic disease, we ask: Where is the 'self'? We suggest that self-agency is lost in this process (Koch et al., 2004). As Reason (1998) argues, 'any internal capacity they may have for intentionally augmenting and cultivating their self-healing capacity is effectively ruled out by the dominant paradigm'. Persons are not allowed to participate in the development of their own well-being. We constitute part of the movement within health care to reverse this, and to make patient participation the core of health practices, hence the appeal of human flourishing at individual and community levels. At the same time we are cognizant of power relations operating in every phase of the participatory action research process. We observe and record its effects. We also reflect on our own role as facilitators and engage in dialogue with the research team about our various positions.

Exploration of power relations

We can explore power relations on three levels (Reason, 1998). The first power level involves the capacity to directly influence events. This may include the involvement of the person who lives with an illness in decisions concerning their care. At this level we may accept things as taken for granted because there appears to be no alternative. People attempting to have a voice about their care are likely to be seen as difficult and as non-compliant.

Second level power may allow the participants to influence the agenda in health care; here a client may be involved in making decisions about a range of possible treatments, including alternative therapies previously excluded from medicine's treatment agenda. Someone attempting to exercise this level of power within an authoritative health knowledge framework is likely to be seen as misinformed.

On a third power level, the person and/or community recognizes power relations and questions authority. With this realization, viewpoints can be reframed to suit emerging situations. Other people's perspectives are recognized as significant and valuable. Reason (1998, pp. 147–167) argues that this leads 'inevitably to a deeply democratic attitude and to participative behaviour toward others'. This ability to inquire into and make sense of our world is available to us all but thrives only in a supportive nurturing environment. Capacity building becomes an active ingredient of participatory action. We subscribe to Freire's (1970) view that capacity can be built though wise, loving and liberating education that nurtures its evolution. However, we need to be cautious, as within the dominant medical perspectives those people questioning its knowledge frameworks are rendered 'insane' (Reason, 1998).

Capacity building with people inevitably leads to confronting authority. 'Expert' patients who question the authority of their medical practitioner are treated with suspicion. Participants have found some responses to verge on hostility. Participants need skills to both grow and be sustained in these confrontational environments. There are practical and moral issues to be discussed within the participatory action research process. We concur with Reason (1998) that the challenge is to design institutions that manifest valid forms of democratic principles, and to find ways in which they can be maintained in self-correcting and creative tension.

In the following section Debbie Kralik writes reflectively about her role as a facilitator.

Email conversations with men and women who have chronic illness

Kralik has been the facilitator of a longitudinal study that has generated data via an online collaborative inquiry group. In this section she shares some of her reflections whilst researching.

Longitudinal research with men and women learning to live with chronic illness is in progress, where the aim is to explicate transition, that is, the way in which people can 'move on' and incorporate the consequences of illness into their lives (Kralik, 2002). Conversations between men and women (in separate gender groups) have taken place daily from July 2003 until 2005 using a facilitated, private electronic mail (email) discussion list (Kralik et al., 2006).

The decision to utilize email as a method for generating longitudinal research data developed from our understanding of the consequences of illness that people living with chronic conditions confront in their lives. Fatigue, pain, social withdrawal and decreased mobility pose challenges to these people that may limit their involvement in research that utilized data generation via group or one to one interviews. Engaging in daily email conversations has created building blocks of text that reveal rich life stories, which when analysed will further explicate the experience of incorporating a long term illness into daily life.

The Internet or World Wide Web (WWW) enables people with computers to communicate with each other. We recognized the potential of using email to enable discussion between research participants (Kralik et al., 2006). It has also been a useful approach for both data generation and data management because we have been able to read, reply, print, forward or file extended messages that have been electronically transmitted (Mann & Stewart, 2000). The use of email has enabled data generation and analysis to occur concurrently, and has provided the means for us to research alongside people living with chronic illness and describe the process of transition through illness (Kralik, 2002). We have developed a web site that includes more detailed information about the background to the research: http://www.unisa.edu.au/nur/arc_project/

A learning circle

The group conversational processes have developed into a 'learning circle', which has fed into the cycle of action learning operationalized as 'look, think and act'. Learning circles are virtual communities that have no fixed locations or time zones and have been an effective and practical method of learning and social change (Hiebert, 1996). Community organizations, trade unions, churches and social justice groups have used learning circles to empower their members to make choices and take action. The distinctions between a learning circle and a discussion group are that learning circles are more focused than a discussion group, are based on common resources and are intended to have action outcomes.

Story telling is privileged to a great extent in this type of online community discussion. The story told online, however, is only part of the story. A story line continues to evolve in the life of the participant as a direct result of reflecting on either the sent or received information. The virtual and real life situations become inseparable.

A learning circle involves groups of people who discuss issues of importance to them and society. They learn at their own pace, reflecting on their own experiences and understandings, without a lecturer or an expert 'running the show'. A researcher facilitates the group conversations by asking questions, prompting reflection and providing alternate ways of thinking. Participants set the agenda for discussion by identifying the issues that are important to them. Learning how to live with long term illness is not just preparation for life, it is a way of life for group members. Exchanging ideas and experiences enhances learning because it is inherently a social process of constructing shared understandings. The facilitated groups provide structure and process to the learning circle and create a shared way of understanding.

The 'action' has not always been as obvious due to constraints such as pain and mobility; however, participants are able to make sense of their experiences (sense making is often the act). Clearly, when we make sense of our experiences through the reflection processes of looking and thinking, possibilities for action become ignited. Developing these online communities has been about creating a shared way of thinking about our world and ourselves.

Reflection in action

The cycles of reflection and action are integral to this collaborative inquiry. In this research, reflection has flowed naturally within the discussions. The use of email has provided the participants with the time to reflect and make sense of their experiences prior to communicating to the group and hence enabled rich data to emerge. Bray et al. (2000) described the three forms of reflection as being descriptive, evaluative and practical. Descriptive reflection relates to responses to the discussions experienced by the group. In this group, descriptive reflection has occurred continuously. Evaluative reflection critiques actions, thoughts and feelings, as related to the inquiry process. The group engaged in evaluative reflection when discussing their responses to each other, how they felt about the inquiry process, and how they felt about being a part of the group. Practical reflection occurs when a summary of the conversations is given as feedback to the group, and in project team meetings when decisions regarding continuation of the project have been made.

Storytelling has been central to the group discussions, particularly because communication by email has removed the dimensions of body language, tone of voice and facial expression that face to face communication provides. Bray et al. (2000) noted that storytelling is particularly valuable when working with diverse groups. The participants in the on-line groups range in age from 25 to 68 years, have diverse medical diagnosis and reside in diverse geographical areas (urban, rural and remote). Storytelling has been effective as the starting point for the making of meaning in the experiences of the participants.

The aim of collaborative inquiry is to construct meaningful, practical knowledge from the experiences of the participants. The group process enables enriched insights into the experiences of others, so that the group can find meaning in these experiences. Collaborative, reflective discussions are helpful in generating deeper insights and understandings. This inquiry has generated data that have been transformed into knowledge through using reflections on the similarities and differences between participants' experiences.

Facilitation and reflection

Self-reflection is a requirement of the participatory action research process but it can be difficult for researchers to make known our assumptions, presuppositions and choices. Disclosure often means sharing one's own experiences with the group. We research in the awareness that our history and the various communities to which we belong influence our interpretations. Journaling and analysing the way in which our horizon is operating is important whilst researching. During this longitudinal research, Kralik uses prompts to aid reflection:

- Do the words I use betray my attitudes to topics?
- What unintended outcomes do I bring about through my own facilitation style?
- Have I self-authorized the facilitation role that I have taken on?
- Is control in these conversations important and why?
- Do I confuse 'facilitation' with 'control'?
- How do I know that I am not projecting my own importance onto this group?
- Can I consciously replace control with trust?
- Can I be present and in connection with others?
- Can I be vulnerable and have a 'don't know' mind, and thereby be open to new learning?
- Can I invite ambiguity and uncertainty to enter the conversations?

Asking these questions during the research process will focus attention on interpretation and facilitate our own reflection. These questions continue to prompt my thinking about contexts and how they affect judgements and interpretations.

The participants in the email groups have challenged us as researchers to reflect upon our definitions of both participation and facilitation.

It has become evident that facilitation in a longitudinal project such as this is a challenging and artful role. The groups have become self-aware through reflection without being driven, probed or 'controlled' by a researcher. However, we are conversing with the participants over a long period of time and constant self-reflection can be exhausting and/or boring, so lighter times are also needed. We have learnt to trust the cyclic nature of using 'look, think and act' within the learning circle and consequently we have identified shifts in understandings that have occurred over time in conversations on the same topic. Learning to live with chronic illness needs time, and we have learnt to respect that need for time so that through reflection action may occur.

Dealing with discord

Discord or conflict can be anticipated as not every person has developed the skills to participate in a group. Discord is a disagreement resulting from individuals or groups that differ in attitudes, beliefs, values or needs. It can also originate from past rivalries or perceptions of difference. Conflict may also arise when people perceive that their needs or the needs of the group are not being met. People may perceive differences in the severity, causes and consequences of the issues being focused upon.

Conflicts can arise when people try to make others change their actions or try to gain an unfair advantage. Values are beliefs or principles we consider to be very important. Serious conflicts arise when people hold incompatible values or when values are not clear. When one party refuses to accept that the other party holds something as a value rather than a preference, the result is most likely to be discord. Conflict can also occur when people ignore their own or others' feelings and emotions or when feelings and emotions differ over a certain issue.

Power relations as discussed earlier can be a cause for discord within groups. Developing and regularly reviewing and revising group norms or ways of working together can help to counter conflict. Participatory action research is about bringing people together for a period of engagement; it is about learning to listen and hear the voices of others. The root of conflict is often that people feel they have not been heard (Boxes 7.1 and 7.2).

Conflict is not always negative; in fact, it is sometimes an impetus for change. When conflict situations are effectively facilitated, they can lead to growth, innovation and new ways of thinking. A participative process may actively resolve conflict. If the feelings underlying a conflict situation are understood, it may be possible for parties to reach consensus that meets both the individual's and the community's needs. This results in mutual benefits and strengthens relationships. If

---

Box 7.1 Group norms for an email participatory action research group.

- Make sure your email is addressed to the list because we all want to know what you have to say.
- Include information relevant to what you are writing about in the subject line.
- Be good listeners (or readers) without judging others. If someone states something, we should all read it and not condemn him/her for his/her ideas and thoughts. Support and inclusion of everyone within the group is very important.
- Ensure the mails from the list remain confidential. Always ensure the privacy of group members. What is said within the group stays in the group.
- Refrain from advertising or promoting products or services to others within the group. If unsure, check with the group first.

Box 7.2 Group norms for a face to face participatory action research group.

- Be good listeners without judging others. Support and inclusion of everyone within the group is very important.
- One person speaks at a time. Wait for the other person to finish speaking before you start.
- Be mindful that other people who want to speak should have the opportunity to do so.
- Ensure the privacy of group members. What is said within the group stays in the group.
- Refrain from advertising or promoting products or services to others within the group. If unsure, check with the group first.

---

conflicts are not able to be resolved, at least they have been made visible and parties may agree to disagree.

It is useful to understand what participants' needs are. It is always important to ask group members what they want to gain or achieve from participating in the group. This is one way of setting the agenda for the issues that the group may address. Check with group participants regularly about their perceptions of the group progress. Talk about issues before they reach a level of conflict and talk about ways to address the issues presented.

8 Ethical Considerations

Codes of conduct for research have been developed since 1945. The most well known include the Nuremberg Code (1947), the Declaration of Geneva (1948, 1994), the Resolution on Human Rights (1990, 1995), the Declaration of Helsinki V (1964, 1996) and the Belmont Report (1979). Throughout the world, research bodies have developed and revised ethics guidelines for the undertaking of research. These documents have been developed to prevent the abuse of people participating in research (Hudson, 1999).

There are no rigid rules that will capture the subtlety of ethical situations that arise during research; however, there are some ethical principles for the protection of participants. These principles are known as autonomy, beneficence and justice (Beauchamp & Childress, 2001). Respect for autonomy requires that people be treated as autonomous agents and affirms that people with diminished autonomy be entitled to protection. This principle is reflected in the process of informed consent, where the risks and benefits of involvement in research are disclosed to the potential participant. Beneficence relates to the maximization of possible benefits for the participant while minimizing possible harm that may result from involvement in the research. One of the areas of ethical difficulty for researchers has been to determine what harm is, and how far it is reasonable to protect people from the often unforeseeable kinds of harm that may follow from their participation in a research project.

The third principle, justice, seeks a fair distribution of the burdens and benefits associated with research so that certain individuals or groups do not bear disproportionate risks while others reap the benefits. It is our perception that when a researcher emphasizes the importance of making a helpful contribution to the person or group being studied, many, if not all, of the other ethical responsibilities also are fulfilled. However, participatory action research is a complex process and whilst often we can anticipate ethical issues that may arise and prepare for their resolution, occasionally we have been caught in dilemmas.

Many of the ethical dilemmas that have confronted us during participatory action research inquiries have been relational ethics or ethics that are situated in a relationship. Relational ethics is based on the premise that 'human experience is, in principle, shared experience' (Macmurray, 1961, p. 61). Core elements essential to relational ethics include: 'mutual respect, engagement, embodied knowledge, uncertainty or possibility and attention to the environment' (Austin et al., 2003, p. 47). Relational ethics emerges from the understanding that we are inter-dependent upon each another. Our world is shaped by the way others respond to us. Ethical action starts with understanding the other's perspective and vulnerability, which requires authentic engagement between participant and researcher (Austin et al., 2003). 'The uncertainty inherent in human existence is acknowledged and should be embraced' (Austin et al., p. 47). The importance of emotion and feeling in relational ethics is acknowledged and is why this approach fits so well with participatory action research principles.

Proposed research must always deal with ethical considerations. A formally constituted ethics committee will review the proposal and may request clarification of the research processes from the researchers or further information to appease their concerns. Formal preparation aside, we will now share with you the ethical issues that arose in this particular study and in so doing provide two practical demonstrations of the participatory action research process. One inquiry explored sexuality with women who had multiple sclerosis. The other was a feminist participatory inquiry that incorporated the use of correspondence (email and letter writing) with midlife women during a 12 month period to learn how they incorporated chronic illness into their lives (Kralik et al., 2000; Kralik, 2002).

Women living with multiple sclerosis

The inquiry we have selected for exploration of ethical issues aimed to understand how 12 women who live with multiple sclerosis (MS) experienced changes to their sexuality. Women living with MS and their particular focus on sexuality provided the canvas to explore (with them) the construction of sexuality and the ways sexuality shapes their lives. We inquired about the relationship between self-identity and the body and observed the transitions that occur as a result of living with MS. These observations may further our understanding about the experience of transition when living with chronic illness. Women who had participated in our previous inquiries (Kralik, Koch & Telford, 2001a; Eastwood et al., 2002; Koch et al., 2002) had raised sexuality as an important issue for them, so we sought and received funding to research with women living with MS. The research was granted ethics approval only after the researcher was asked to address the ethics committee. It seems that the word 'sexuality' sparked some apprehension. Concerns raised by members of the ethics committee included that the inquiry had the potential to alter the lives of women's partners. Discussion focused on the notion of sexuality being a part of life, and to ignore the changes that women with MS experience in their sexuality would be a greater ethical issue. The committee was satisfied that we were sensitive to the possibility that the impact of the research would go beyond just the participants attending the group.

The women joined us for the first few meetings and group norms were articulated and agreed upon by the group. These included openness, honesty and the keeping of all conversations in confidence.

The first ethical issue raised here is that we cannot predict what will be revealed during participatory action research meetings, and while we aim to create a strong, supportive, safe environment, there may be times when harm threatens. This is where the elements of relational ethics become profoundly important. Story telling was commenced; each woman in turn talked about sexuality in her life and researchers also disclosed the meaning of sexuality for them. During the first few group meetings we listened to each other respectfully. One woman told her story about being sexually abused as a child. The story describing a child being violated, beaten and abused shocked some of us. Being mindful that research should do no harm, it was important to ascertain that everyone was comfortable with these proceedings.

We were assured that whilst some women were horrified at the frank disclosures, it was sobering for them learn that sexual beginnings have the power to shape subsequent sexual responses. They revealed feeling fortunate that their sexual histories had been less complicated. Meanwhile the woman who told the story of abuse had told it many times before in the effort to 'move on' from her childhood of abuse. The pain associated with disclosure had dulled through the retelling and on this occasion she had felt validated by others in the group through their expressed concern.

While we cannot predict what will be revealed in participatory action research groups, we can predict that someone in the group will have a louder voice than others. Power relations may be at play here and as facilitators we have strategies for guiding louder participants. For example, the progressive nature of MS had made one woman forgetful. The same story was repeated at regular intervals and this became a group irritant. The ethical issue here is that every one has a right to be heard, but how does a facilitator sensitively address repetitions? The researchers met with Jo (fictional) afterwards and explained the situation to her. She was aware that she often repeated herself; hence, we agreed that one of us would raise a hand visibly to remind Jo that she was repeating herself. When shrouded in good-natured humour, this simple strategy appeared to work most of the time.

Another ethical issue arose when one woman revealed that she did not believe privacy within the group had been upheld. She met with us after a group meeting to say that she perceived that information had been leaked. Given the topic for conversation was sexuality, Sue (a fictional name) felt unsafe with disclosing further information during group meetings.

Our response as researchers was to abort the group meetings and consider other ways of data generation. Instead we offered women the opportunity of one to one interviews to be held in each woman's home. Nine women volunteered to participate in the interviews. This allowed us to gain additional in-depth data about individual experiences and ensured confidentiality. Interview questions sought to explore self and identity and transition. The interviews were like conversations where the participant led direction and flow. We made an assumption that the conversations about living with MS were about those aspects of life that were important to the women. Their constructions were an interpretation of life and were influenced by pre-understandings (fore-understandings), experience, language, culture, generation/age, education, gender and socio-political knowledge. The challenge was to maintain a balance between flexibility and consistency in data generation. One to one interviews were recorded, transcribed and analysed. Each woman interviewed also received her own analysed story for her input and changes were made as requested. We believe it is an ethical decision that people have a right to their own stories.

Themes identifying common claims, issues and concerns were identified across interviews. It was then time to convene participatory action research group meetings to discuss commonalities. Talking about common aspects of sexuality rather than individual accounts secured a safe environment for the continuation of the group process. One way to forge the participatory action research process is to talk about common experiences. Subsequent actions can lead to the reforms envisaged.

Earlier we said that individual stories were given to each woman for their input and that changes were made as requested. The communal story, describing common issues, claims and concerns was also disseminated to all participants. We advocate using the spoken words of participants in subsequent publications. We ask that each participant pay attention to the way their voice is recorded, and we assess whether they are concerned about voice identification even if fictional names are used. All stakeholders receive a printout of papers published.

It came as a surprise when one woman contacted us a year later with her concern about being identified in the published paper. Whilst she had signed off on the copy for publication, she had changed her mind. She was involved in a legal situation with her ex-husband and she did not want one aspect of her story identified. Clearly it was too late for us to respond to this situation.

Constructions of sexuality encompassed physical sexual responses, perceptions of appearance and attractiveness to self and others, communication and relationships, self-image and self-esteem, and the sense of affirmation and acknowledgment that women experienced from others in their everyday lives. It came to our attention that one woman, Jan, was very unhappy in her relationship. She described being sexually taken when her husband had a desire for sex. Wheelchair bound and incontinent she believed that these unwanted sexual encounters were the only validation she had of being a person. In one of the last participatory action research group sessions she told the group that she had attempted to commit suicide. The women came to her immediate support and surprised her with their strong affirmation of her as a person. Researching with people who are suffering can be emotionally overwhelming, but being present with them often helps to alleviate the suffering, even if only for a short time. As researchers we felt it was important to follow this through. Our ethical response was to discuss Jan's situation with community health services that were already closely assisting her. Whilst not disclosing Jan's discussion within the group, we did strongly suggest the need for close monitoring and care. Unforeseen ethical dilemmas can occur in any inquiry; however, it is the role of the researcher and research team to respond in a sensitive way. A relational ethics approach values personhood, engagement and connection with others. Sometimes an ethical action is to just 'be there' for others because relational ethics is about being with others as well as being for the other (Austin et al., 2003).

Women with chronic illness

Ethical behaviours in participatory research are a dynamic, practical and interpersonal activity, and may depend on striking a fine balance between the rights of the participants, the risk of exploitation and the wider purposes of the research (Price, 1996; Seymour & Ingleton, 1999). Qualitative research can reveal difficult and hidden issues in an insightful way and often these issues confront us ethically. Often the process of resolution of an ethical issue is just as important as the outcome. In the section to follow Kralik shares some of the ethical considerations and lessons learnt during a participatory study that involved corresponding (letter or email) for one year with 81 women who were learning to live with chronic illness (Kralik, 2002). The aim of the study was to understand the experiences of midlife women living with chronic illness. The excerpt in Box 8.1 shows that people

Box 8.1 'The poster girl for fearful friends' by Trish.

My husband rarely saw me cry. I come from the type of family with the school of thought real people only cry into their pillows and certainly don't burden others. Hmmm . . . all bets went off on that one when my husband and I were both diagnosed with cancer in the same week.

I had that need to be strong for a poor sick man. He was incidentally diagnosed with renal cell cancer while in the hospital with pneumonia. At the same time I am seeing my GP and getting a mammogram then rushed off to see a surgeon. It was a bad week. I wailed, in the car, on sidewalks, home alone in bed, in elevators, again and again. I cried like he had died already. At that point, I didn't mind if mine were terminal or not, but no way was I sticking around without my man. I mourned him. Both of us have a good prognosis. Both of us have a 40% chance of recurrence, but I feel this cancer is with me for life.

Chronic illness maybe, but I know that I do have chronic fear. Every woman I know has gone for a mammogram because at 43, I had a mastectomy as a day patient. Maybe there are good uses for some fears. I am a poster girl for fearful friends. 'Will she/won't she make it? Is she telling us the truth? Really telling us the worst? Don't hold back, we can take it'. Friends and family want assurance as much as I do, so I tell them what I can. I tell them everything is lovely and hold my own fears close. It does not seem right to share fears; facts, yes, fears, no.

Oh my, the anger I feel towards my ex-GP and soon-to-be ex-surgeon. That will take some work to let go of. I decided she needed a good kick in her too complacent arse. I have seen her for years and she never gave me a breast exam or suggested a routine mammogram. I wrote her an angry letter so maybe she will be a little more diligent in regards to her other patients. Not a bad doctor, just lax in patient care. I had an excellent doctor before this one, unfortunately retired, but I am not going to have less than an excellent doctor again. I am not going to allow anyone else to bet my life again. As to the surgeon, mediocre and adequate, paternalistic (which to me is inherently obnoxious). God, don't you hate that 'Don't worry your pretty little head about it' attitude? I take that as 'I (the doctor) hate having to explain or reassure'. Worse yet, when they denigrate questions because they know all the answers . . . or would like you to think that.

Most definitely I am angry with myself for succumbing to cancer panic. 'Just cut it off' I said. I remain angry with him for not reassuring me that I had time, for not telling me not to panic, for not telling me to take time to research. I do not regret the mastectomy, just the doctor I let do it. Sloppy work. Haste makes waste is not just an adage. God it's a fact. I spent most of my time researching renal cell cancer and querying my husband's doctor. I ran out of steam or just couldn't cope with looking at my own health stuff. I did do some though, and I did ask my

(Continued)

Box 8.1   *(Continued).*

surgeon if he did sentinel node biopsy. I surely had choices and access to great care. He said sometimes he did, and I let it slide. I wake up with ten nodes gone, and a nerve severed that needn't have been, and this man surgeon doesn't see the big deal? He probably saved my life, right? Maybe, but he made sure I will have to worry about every paper cut or pinprick on my left arm forever. I think it's a shame more men don't get breast cancer, maybe then he could identify and give it another five minutes to do a good job rather than the minimum standard. He did unnecessary damage but that's OK cause he saved my life? What about quality of life too? Am I just too demanding? I don't think so. Lord I fought and bitched and got my husband the best possible care and made sure he suffered no complications or side-effects from an 'adequate' doctor or overworked staff. God I wish I had someone to look out for me the same way when I was down and out. Angry is it for now. Most of my friends find me amusing, charming, and entertaining as always. Most don't know of the anger. I guess the anger will work itself out eventually.

come to participatory inquiry from diverse past experiences and often with complex and different agendas.

If we were to interpret this story guided by the work of Frank (1995), we could say that Trish has displaced fear of contingency into anger and has turned on others. Whilst her anger can be justified, and as readers we can be outraged on her behalf, the ethical issue here is that we would like to help her move on but we are not quite sure how to proceed. She is living a story of chaos and the immediate impulse is to advance some therapy, perhaps achieved through acknowledging her story. But Frank (1995, p. 110) reminds us that chaos is 'never transcended but must be accepted before new lives can be built and new stories told'. Accordingly it may be harmful to an individual if a health professional rushes someone to move on. While it is under-stood that moving on is desirable, we are reminded that chaos is the 'pit of narrative wreckage'. We are conscious about the anxiety that the chaos story provokes in others in the health care team. But attempting to push the person out of this wreckage compounds the chaos. It often leads to labelling the person, or worse, the person is dismissed or labelled with depression or as being 'in denial'. When we invite story telling there are potential ethical consequences. The point being made here is that the invitation to tell one's story means acknowledging that there may be ethical consequences.

There have been some broad assumptions made that qualitative methods are inherently less potentially harmful than other forms of research conducted in health care settings (Faulkner, 1980; Field, 1989;

DeRenzo, 1998; Seymour & Ingleton, 1999). This assumption may lead to an under-examination of issues that emerge as a result of the intense relationships that develop during the participatory action research process. Such issues may be difficult to resolve and potentially damaging to both the participant and the researcher (Guba & Lincoln, 1989; De Raeve, 1994; Seymour & Ingleton, 1999).

In this study, it was important that I understood the need for ethical sensitivity and the potentially exploitative nature of this research. The women were vulnerable and I was aware that they had entrusted me with intimate information. The writing up of the report entailed grappling with the issue of anonymity, specifically the extent to which this could be preserved. I came to understand that anonymity must be negotiated between us (the women and the researcher) just as issues of consent were constantly negotiated during the 12 month period of data generation. The women needed to read how they were portrayed in the final report before they could make decisions about the degree of anonymity that they desired. The reliance on natural language and the use of direct quotes, which contribute to 'rich descriptions' in qualitative research, means that individual anonymity can be difficult to uphold (Ford & Reutter, 1990; Seymour & Ingleton, 1999). I excluded any information that might expose the woman's identity and I used pseudonyms for all women in the final report that I distributed to each woman who had been involved. Once women read the report, they could decide if changes needed to be made. Many women wrote that they could identify themselves and most women indicated that they would like their pseudonym changed to their real name. Several participants wrote that they no longer have anything to hide and that they were proud of their involvement in the study and wished to use their real name. With humour, Beverley wrote:

'I would like to use my real name in the paper. It was funny when I first read the paper, I was thinking "Gee that Bronwyn sounds just like me, how amazing", then of course it clicked. I am slow off the mark some days!'

Disengagement

The issue of disengagement from the women who participated in this research was perceived as an ethical issue. Disengagement is the state that researchers achieve when they finish their research and 'leave the field'. This is always difficult when relationships have been formed and participants perceive they have benefited from being involved in the research. In this study I became aware that disengagement from some women who participated in the study might be an issue. They had enjoyed the reciprocity and writing of their stories and reading the experiences of other women, which seemed to mirror their own. Now the dialogic process was over. It was necessary to reduce the amount of time I was spending writing letters and emails, in order to proceed with the inquiry.

I started to distance myself from the women with a card and letter that thanked them for their involvement. I took the time to hand write each card with a personal message. I wanted each woman to feel she had made a valuable contribution to the research. It was not an easy process to begin to disengage because of the way in which we had journeyed together. I had been immersed in their lives and we had developed close relationships. I used empathy, tact and diplomacy to leave the relationships that had been established.

When the women joined the study they were aware that our pen pal relationship was for the purposes of research. Since closure of the study, many women have continued to intermittently write to me to provide an update on their progress or events in their lives. These are social letters and I take pleasure in receiving them. At the time of closure, I received many thank you notes from the women for the opportunity to tell their story. Letters came from the husband of one woman and the brother of another woman. They wrote to tell me of the positive changes that they had noticed in their partner or sister, which they attributed to involvement in the study.

The close relationships we developed made disengagement difficult for some women, because they had used me as a listening post. In some instances, the women used their writings and involvement in the research for therapeutic reasons. An example was when Rhondda wrote of a secret she had never told anyone, but she felt the secret was the reason she had developed cancer. She felt it was time to tell her secret as a way of letting 'go of some of this baggage' that she had been carrying around for a large part of her life. I was concerned that she was giving away parts of herself that she may later regret – parts of herself that went outside the purpose of our research. I wrote that:

'This secret does not need to be divulged for the purposes of our research. You are free to write what you wish, and you know that I will always listen and offer you support in any way I can, but please understand that I do not need to know the secret to understand your experiences of living with cancer.'

Rhondda chose to tell her secret, writing that she had unloaded so many of her painful experiences onto paper and had felt better for it. She felt that telling her secret might have a similar feeling:

'I am actually surprised I am enjoying this whole exercise, even at times when it has meant bearing the soul and having to resurface deep buried thoughts and painful experiences. I (have) gained a lot of comfort getting feelings onto paper and off my chest. I felt once I had written them down, they were dealt with in some form.'

I had guessed what her secret was before she wrote it as she had given me clues in her writings. I knew that it was an immense burden that she carried, and had eroded her self-esteem over the years. Even though I had promised confidentiality, I felt considerable responsibility as keeper of this secret. I never referred to the secret in a direct way in my writings to her, fearful that a member of her family may read the email before she did. Rhondda has continued to keep in touch.

Throughout the research process, I found that my attempts to establish ground rules or principles about what made me as a researcher too close, or too disconnected, became absurd. Through reflection on the research process, I can see that the changes many of us experienced meant that it is our narratives of connection that had significance. Who we are is in constant change, and that includes our ability to understand and be understood by others.

This research had a period of crisis towards the end of the dialogic process. The development of a web site had been enjoyable for those who had been involved, and the women were very proud of their achievement. They visited the web site regularly to read each other's stories and the posts left by visitors. On one such visit that Rhondda made to the web site, she decided to visit one of the web rings our web site was linked to. With uncanny timing, only 2 days following revealing her life long secret to me, she was greeted with satanic messages. The web ring had been 'hacked' with satanic messages that were only present for a short time. Rhondda was shattered, perceiving that she had disclosed her deepest self to a satanist. She thought I had targeted her after reading about her 'devious ways'. She kept her fears to herself for 3 days, tearful and barely sleeping, before she made contact with an associate researcher who then contacted me and also continued to remain in contact with Rhondda. Links with all web rings were immediately severed, but the healing for Rhondda was not so easy:

> 'I am so devastated and couldn't comprehend why you would do this to me. I also felt we had a special pen pal relationship; I valued your opinions, felt totally confident in trusting you. I did feel I had been betrayed. One thing the study has helped me with is not bottling things up, get them out in the open, my first thoughts were to change my email address, get a silent phone number and never speak to you again, just drop out. That was the old me. Not confront issues but I am glad I have, the pain will ease, and I have been through worse than this and survived.'

Rhondda did not sleep well for days and contacted a counsellor at her place of employment. As a researcher, I was deeply distressed that through the process of this research, someone had been harmed, a woman with whom a close relationship had developed. Rhondda lived interstate, hence I sent an email sincerely apologizing and explaining that I was not aware that the web ring had been hacked:

> 'I am so very sorry to have hurt you. I have learnt a tremendous lesson . . . once again you are the teacher. I have learnt not to be naive. It never occurred to me in my wildest dreams that the links would be used in that way. This experience has reiterated just how careful, very careful, I must be with the people who trust me. Not only in this study but the others I am involved with as well. I thank you for giving me the opportunity to explain. I will leave it to you whether you would like your story removed, and your involvement ceased. I will also destroy all our correspondence should you request it.'

We sent many emails to each other, with the aim of understanding the events that had taken place. Rhondda talked with her relatives who were experienced with computers and web sites. They assured her that hacking of web sites is a 'common occurrence'. Rhondda wrote to me:

> 'I do believe you to be innocent D . . . , I have cried buckets, not slept, not attended medical appointments, not left the house. I am 3 days behind in Christmas preparations, have not attended to the volunteer work that was entrusted to me. Have made myself sick with grief, that is the only way to describe what this has felt like, like going through bereavement, only I haven't worked through all the stages yet. The web can be a dangerous place as we have both discovered. I too, have learnt a lot.'

Rhondda came to believe that I was innocent of being involved in the hacking and slowly we rebuilt our relationship, and perhaps the experience provided an even greater understanding of each other. With the help of Rhondda's adult children, who joked with their mother about our crisis, we have also come to make the occasional joke about that experience.

Having revisited my crisis with Rhondda, I learnt that the most significant issue for me as the researcher was that I was physically distanced from the women who may be experiencing emotional pain, and this must be considered as a significant ethical issue when using correspondence to generate sensitive data. At the beginning of our inquiry, when contact was first made with each woman, I had established where and what her support systems were and had also obtained a contact phone number and address for her general medical practitioner. There were times, however, when the distance between us concerned me.

The literature offers little guidance for researchers inquiring on sensitive subjects where participants are at risk of psychological distress. Nurse researchers insist that qualitative inquiry should not harm participants (Cowles, 1988; Erlandson et al., 1993; Estroff, 1995;

Munhall, 1988; Smith, 1992; Price, 1996) and have identified some of the risks inherent in qualitative research. However, few researchers have documented their experiences and participants' experiences of researching on sensitive subjects. This is unfortunate because the documentation of such accounts may be useful for other qualitative researchers. Participatory action researchers hear many stories but their own are equally important and should also be conveyed.

When using correspondence to generate data, the researcher must rely on the participant to describe her feelings as well as her experiences. Kavanaugh and Ayres (1998) suggest that looking at decontextualized comments made by a participant may mislead the researcher. This advice is made more complex when communicating by correspondence, because it can be difficult for the researcher to understand the emotion that has accompanied the disclosure.

There were women who wrote during times when they were obviously depressed and I found it difficult to gauge their intent through writing. It was difficult to evaluate the woman's response to the telling of her story through correspondence. The reduced availability of social cues when using correspondence was an issue that needed to be considered. Although I never contacted a family member or doctor because of my concerns for a woman, I came very close to taking this action when Sandra wrote:

> 'I am ready to drive off the edge of a freeway bridge. I had never felt so entirely crushed in my entire and total life. I was transformed from being an adult to being a 4-year-old child . . . I felt utterly vulnerable, utterly weird, and utterly useless.'

To further complicate matters, Sandra lived in another country. I kept in close contact with her as she continued to write of her distress about being victimized at her place of employment because of her disability. Sandra was a professional person, and recognized her reaction to this situation as impacting on her life in a significant way and sought counselling. She had lived many years with her disabilities, including a facial disability, but she had been shattered by some thoughtless remarks made by a person in the hierarchy at her work. It was not long following this incident that she was able to change her work place.

The gradual development of a safe and trusting relationship between the women and me was important to allow the women to disclose at their own pace:

> 'I can feel myself shutting up again . . . after exposing myself too much. It's all a bit new . . . and I look forward to your soft letters. That's how they feel to me. This world can be hard and uncaring at times but softness is such a welcomed feeling.'

There were times when women disclosed personal problems to me and I became aware of the need not to offer advice, even though my opinion may have been sought. At first I found it difficult to know how to respond to direct requests for help or advice and tried to divert or avoid these issues.

In these circumstances, I acknowledged the woman's issue and reiterated that she was the teacher and the holder of knowledge. If the issue were relevant to living with a chronic illness, I would ask questions with the aim of understanding the issues. When the woman worked through her responses to these questions, she often viewed her issue with a new clarity.

Summary

When discussing the ethical dilemmas in the two studies cited, we come to see that each ethical situation is unique and that there is no single solution. People's stories that describe their experiences are fundamental to human flourishing and their stories are framed by a background of the interpretations of their experiences.

> 'Ethics makes sense when we engage with it. It is in hearing other people's stories, their values, beliefs, reasons and reasoning, whys and wherefores, that we engage with these things ourselves.'
>
> (Tschudin, 2003, p. 62)

Stories are created to be told and heard. Stories prompt us to think and can promote understanding, and change the actions of individuals and communities. Often when researching with people using participatory action research principles, the ethical situations that arise exist because we are relational beings:

> 'Ethical behaviour is not the display of one's moral rectitude in times of crisis . . . it is the day-to-day expression of one's commitment to other persons and the ways in which human beings relate to one another in their daily interactions.'
>
> (Levine, 1977, p. 846)

Relational ethics from researchers using participatory action research principles means initiating and maintaining conversations, and more than that, it means that ethics is found in our daily obligations and the way we respond to one another.

9 Development of Community Partnerships

Co-authored by Dr Anne van Loon and Dr Susan Mann

Outside the field of chronic illness experience we have applied our theoretical understanding of transition in capacity building programmes or community development. Story telling and reclaiming self-identity is part of that work (Gergen, 1991; Kleinman, 1998; Kelly & Field, 1996; Nettleton & Watson, 1998; Brody, 2003). Further, a book published by Penguin in 2005 explores transition with 24 centenarians (Koch et al., 2005). We were interested to hear stories of transition throughout the lifespan so we travelled across Australia to interview 24 dynamic older people. Community-based participatory research in health is a collaborative approach to research that equitably involves all partners in the research process and recognizes the unique strengths that each brings. 'Community participatory action research begins with a research topic of importance to the community with the aim of combining knowledge and action for social change to improve community health' (Minkler & Wallerstein, 2003, p. 4).

Participatory action methods are now increasingly used in the development of community health organizational partnerships. These projects put participation, action research and adult education at the forefront of attempts to liberate and emancipate disempowered people. Participatory action methods are being used not only so that local people can inform outsiders, but also for people's own analysis of their own situations and conditions. Participatory action is particularly prevalent in projects regarding farm sustainability, livelihood improvement and natural resource management. To the wider body of development programmes, projects and initiatives, participatory action approaches represent a significant departure from historical and standard practices.

Israel et al. (1998) proposed the following key principles of community-based research, which are widely accepted in the field of public health.

(1) *Recognizes community as a unit of identity.* This research should work explicitly with communities, which may be defined by a geographical area, or defined as a community of identity that is geographically dispersed but whose members hold a sense of

common identity and shared fate. The focus is on cumulative learning by all the participants and, given the nature of these approaches as systems of inquiry, their use has to be participative.

(2) *Builds on strengths and resources within the community.* This research should explicitly identify, support and reinforce social structures, processes and knowledge already existing in the community that help participants work together to improve their lives.

(3) *Facilitates collaborative partnerships in all phases of the research.* This research should involve community members in every phase they want to participate in, including but not limited to: issue definition, data collection, interpretation of results, and application of the results to address community concerns. This may involve applying skills from outside the community, but should focus on issues identified by the community and create situations in which all parties can truly influence the entire research process.

(4) *Integrates knowledge and action for mutual benefit of all partners.* Though the research project itself might not include a direct action component, all parties must have a commitment to applying the research results to a social change effort intended to benefit all partners.

(5) *Promotes a co-learning and empowering process that attends to social inequalities.* This research should recognize the inherent inequalities between marginalized communities and researchers, and attempt to address these by emphasizing knowledge of community members and sharing information, resources and decision-making powers. Israel et al. offer the example that researchers learn from the knowledge and local theories of the community members, and community members acquire further skills in how to conduct research.

(6) *Involves a cyclical and iterative process.* This research should involve trust building, partnership development and maintenance in all phases of the research.

(7) *Disseminates findings and knowledge gained to all partners.* This research should disseminate information gained in a respectful and understandable language that acknowledges all participants' contributions and ownership of the knowledge production.

The capability of a participatory action research approach to acknowledge diversity and complexity in community partnership is considered a strength. The assumption is that different individuals and groups make different evaluations of situations, which lead to different actions. All views of activity or purpose are context specific and rich with interpretation, bias and prejudice. Clearly, the focus is on cumulative and collaborative learning by all involved in the project. The participatory action approach in the community setting is concerned with actions that will bring about changes that people in the situation regard as improvements. The role of the researchers or project manager is that of assisting people in the context of their situation to undertake their own study about an issue that is important to them, and so achieve meaningful change. The participatory action process leads to consideration and debate about possibilities for meaningful and contextual change. Placing an issue under the spotlight for deliberation and debate often results in the changed perceptions of all involved and a readiness to contemplate action. The action usually includes local community building or strengthening, thereby increasing the capacity of people to initiate sustainable action on their own.

In the following section we share two capacity building inquiries; in the first we researched alongside Australian Aboriginal elders (Project Manager Dr Susan Mann) and in the second we researched with homeless women (Project Manager Dr Anne van Loon).

Look, think and act: researching with Australian Aboriginal elders

'I personally did not understand the seriousness of this affliction until years later, this is when I saw what it was doing to my sister. First her toes were amputated and then up to her knees and then her other leg received that same treatment; in my mind I still see the anguish and pain that she was going through. One day she said to me, "Could you give me that cream cake?" and I replied that wouldn't it be bad for her and I can still hear her reply. "I just do not care any more". My beautiful sister was giving up the fight to live. This still haunts me; it was then that I started to realise what a terrible illness diabetes is.'

One example of the participatory action research process is our work with an Australian indigenous community. Dr Susan Mann was the project manager for this inquiry. 'Diabetes is killing our community' were the words that brought the project manager, the research team and Aboriginal elders together to undertake this study. The Port Lincoln community on the Eyre Peninsula in south Australia has about 600 indigenous Australian people, of whom 200 are reputedly diagnosed with diabetes. The statistics are startling. The death rate related to diabetes is 204% higher for Aboriginal people on the

Eyre Peninsula in comparison with Aboriginal populations in South Australia overall (Nguyen et al., 1996).

Despite the persistent and disproportionate ill health caused by diabetes, the usual medical management approaches have not yielded the necessary improvements for Aboriginal people. Recent reviews have called for more locally responsive participatory programmes that empower Aboriginal people to improve diabetes management (KPMG Management Consulting, 1997; Diabetes Australia, 1998; Kimberley Aboriginal Medical Services Council WA, 1998). This project was funded by the National Health and Medical Research Council and the proposal made its journey through several ethics committees and a Port Lincoln Aboriginal Governance Committee. Approval was granted.

The management of diabetes often involves education for the person diagnosed with diabetes and is underpinned by self-monitoring of metabolic control. Non-adherence with suggested therapeutic regimes is often cited as the most important issue in diabetes management (MacLean & Lo, 1998). Rather than following the medical management route, and leaving behind the controlling language of compliance and non-adherence, we believed greater involvement of Aboriginal families in diabetes management programmes that dealt with issues of concern to them would lead to improved health outcomes. As researchers we proposed that appropriate therapeutic action could be developed collaboratively by Aboriginal families, their health workers and other diabetes educators and clinicians. The value of using empowering approaches to diabetes management has been substantiated by previous research with non-Aboriginal people with type 2 diabetes (Koch, Kralik & Sonnack, 1999; Koch, Kralik & Taylor, 1999). Empowerment in these instances was achieved by skillfully facilitating people towards an exploration of their circumstances, the contexts of their lives, and their experiences with diabetes.

The aim of this 12 month inquiry was twofold: to use participatory action research to improve diabetes self-management with Aboriginal families, and to develop the ability of Aboriginal health workers to use participatory action research. The elders who participated in the project were all residents of Port Lincoln. All belonged to the Council of Aboriginal Elders of South Australia Port Lincoln Forum Incorporated.

When a participatory action research team begins work, it meets with the community and other leaders to ensure that they support the initiative and perceive the potential for their control over the process. Meetings with members of the community are held to describe the process. Separate meetings are also held with specific interest groups (i.e. women, youths, the elderly, and economically active persons) and with individual households. This mixture of public meetings and dialogue with smaller groups makes it more likely that all members of the community will participate constructively.

Looking

Facilitated by Mann, participants were encouraged to talk about their experiences of living with diabetes in response to the following questions: How has diabetes affected your lifestyle? Can you give an example of an incident or episode that really changed your life? How do you feel about what is happening to you? What sorts of things (people or services) help you to manage successfully? Thereafter, the 12 participating elders set the agenda for discussion. Ten sessions or 40 contact hours enabled the opportunity to build trust. People were able to give storied accounts of their experiences. Passing on information and educating others through story telling is well understood within Aboriginal communities. One important realization that emerged from this inquiry is that story telling is a powerful way to make positive changes in people's lives.

Thinking

The group identified four themes that impact on the successful self-management of type 2 diabetes. These themes were: nutrition, better understanding of diabetes, the education of young people, and providing support for family and wider community members. Wrapped around these themes was the need to create a supportive environment where learning can occur. Such learning has the potential to encourage strong and meaningful community action. While understanding of diabetes varied greatly with the group, it was primarily seen as an illness over which individuals had little control. Initially diabetes was seen as debilitating and stopped people doing the activities they wanted to do.

As the group continued to share their experiences, however, the link between nutrition, exercise and medication became more apparent to everyone. One participant found a way to live meaningfully by adjusting her lifestyle and becoming involved on committees. The elders sharing their knowledge in this way resulted in their ability to recognize that their general feeling of wellness could be enhanced with greater understanding of the links between their diet, their physical activity and their medication. The elders also demonstrated generosity and commitment to the education of young people by their willingness to share their time and experiences, especially their experience with alcohol. While they understood that drinking alcohol often had a detrimental effect on their successful management of diabetes, they understood that young people had a great need to belong and that alcohol was one way of feeling included in a group.

Acting

The elders developed a culture within the group that reflected a safe learning environment for all involved. This supportive environment enabled the participants in the group to discuss their fears of either being diagnosed themselves, or having one of their family diagnosed, with diabetes. Initially, they were anxious about what such a diagnosis would mean for themselves and/or their family members. This was expressed in a dominant story of fear, where fear was the controlling factor in their experience of living with diabetes. As fear increased, participants talked about withdrawing from family and friends. Some of the participants blamed God or family.

During the discussions with the group, participants described what it was like to be living with anxiety and fear. This included a fear of doctors, which could lead to anxiety attacks, high blood pressure and increased stress. Living life in this way trapped participants in a way of life that resulted in negativity, depression, and failure to take responsibility for their own health. Fear became the way the group initially described their experiences under the identified themes of nutrition, understanding, education of young people, and support for family and community. Fear therefore became an obstacle to management.

Fear hampered the management of diabetes due to the group's lack of understanding regarding the 'chronic nature' of diabetes. Even when there were many resources available in terms of pamphlets and brochures, participants identified a lack of awareness and education regarding the symptoms of type 2 diabetes. Anxiety and fear prevented them either understanding information or seeking education regarding diabetes. As a result they did not know what diabetes was, they did not understand the link between family history and diabetes, and they did not understand the impact of physical activity on sugar levels. Believing they would 'get over it' they did not attempt to engage in any form of physical activity. Anxiety was increased when available information was conflicting or confusing regarding management of diabetes and the impact of diabetes on lifestyle. Such confusion made keeping up with current knowledge regarding diabetes difficult.

However, in the discussion that followed the elders recognized that they had tackled fear and the way in which they had done this became the topic of conversation. The story that unfolded was one of great courage. The elders discussed ways that they could learn from each other and how their experience could benefit other members of the community. 'Acting' in this context is taking community action.

From fear to courage: creating an alternate community story

As the group progressed and people expressed their fears about diabetes and recognized how fear had dominated and interfered with their management of diabetes, there began to emerge a story of courage that was full of life, creativity, resilience and strength. It is this story of courage that demonstrated how people lived their life in a meaningful way.

Courage enabled people to stand in the face of fear. Courage was recognized in both the person diagnosed with diabetes, and the people caring for or living with a person with diabetes. For the person diagnosed with diabetes, courage was demonstrated by an ability to name fear and accept the diagnosis. This ability was aided through prayer, and support of family and friends. The elders agreed that only when you took responsibility for your own health could you move forwards.

Confidence was increased through the understanding that they were 'not alone' in their experience. Elders recognized and acknowledged their own strengths and felt an enhanced ability to take control of their lives. Their knowledge was affirmed, valued and respected.

Knowledge generated in the group enabled the elders to increase their knowledge and understanding of the impact of diabetes on their life. As their understanding increased, elders gained a greater control and understanding of their choices regarding their health.

Significantly, this group worked towards an elders story day and the production of a booklet telling the stories of their experiences. This outcome was designed to give voice to their experiences in a public forum. The elders story day represented the culmination of their learning and involvement in this project. The booklet *Look, Think, Act: Indigenous Stories about Living with Diabetes* outlined the events as they took place during 2003. The booklet focuses on the voices of the elders as they talk about their life experiences, with a particular focus on their management of type 2 diabetes. They shared their personal experiences of either having diabetes, or caring for a partner and/or family member with diabetes, or wanting to support friends with diabetes. They also discussed their hopes for the future, their hopes for the young, and their plans for rescuing their community from the onslaught of diabetes. Further, the group commenced road shows around the Port Lincoln community. They found that talking about their experience was liberating and they believed this health promotion work was central to their community's development.

Researchers who are also health professionals engaging in the participatory action research process usually undergo a process of attitudinal and behavioural change. They learn to relinquish both power and their role as the expert and enter into a more horizontal form of communication and being with people. This relearning was important for the development of the meaningful actions that were the outcome of this study and the study we describe next.

Capacity building with women who have experienced child sexual abuse and addiction

'Someone told me I was responsible for what I wanted in my life now. That was huge, I didn't even realise that I had a life, let alone that I was responsible for it! I didn't know then . . . I didn't feel or think. I wasn't even in my body most of the time! There was no me.'

This 2 year project, which commenced during August 2003, used the 'look, think, act' model of participatory action research described by Stringer (1999) to work with women survivors of child sexual abuse. Dr Anne van Loon undertook this inquiry. These experiences have led the women to misuse alcohol or illicit drugs/substances, or take up gambling, which has directly contributed to their state of homelessness. Thirteen women connected to an inner city supported accommodation service were voluntarily recruited into the project; thus their willing participation in a group that had the potential for personal growth was likely. Therefore two groups were formed to facilitate a climate that would promote trust, reciprocity and the opportunity for each woman to be heard. The women stated that they were uncomfortable and felt unsafe in a larger group. Dr Anne van Loon, a nurse researcher who was supported by a social worker from the partnering organization, facilitated the two groups. It was anticipated that discussing an abused past could bring up painful memories, which would require counselling support from a trusted worker that the women knew.

Interaction and data generation commenced with an in-depth one to one interview with each woman. She was given the space and time to tell 'her story' of how the sexual abuse experiences had impacted her life, and how and why she came to use/misuse alcohol/drugs/ gambling. These individual stories were analysed and the plot lines of strength and resilience were presented as the starting point for participatory action research group work. Interviews and group meetings used a narrative approach that was audiotaped, transcribed, analysed and given back to the women after each fortnightly participatory action research group for validation, reflection and considered action. Participatory action research groups continued fortnightly cycles for 16 months.

The feedback was presented using verbatim extracts grouped around thematic issues and written up using the 'look, think and act' process to guide reflection. Exemplars from the fortnight's discussion were provided and questions were posited so each woman could systematically name her thoughts and feelings around the issues presented, thus making sense of her own situation and preferred options in relation to that issue, and reflect on which way she might like to move. If possible she should decide what she could do to achieve her desired outcomes. Additionally, findings were summarized and given to two reference groups of service providers ($n = 25$) so that they could reflect on their organizational practice and develop ways to improve services and build capacity and responsiveness to this client group. However, this paper focuses on facilitating reflection in women who participated in the two groups.

Facilitating a trustworthy space for safe reflection

Many adult survivors of child sexual abuse actively repress memories of the events, so they can live and function every day. They avoid discussion of their experiences because it involves disgusting, humiliating and embarrassing details that are painful to recall (Mazza et al., 2001). Their early betrayal and violation make them necessarily suspicious and protective. They have difficulty in trusting people; therefore facilitating group work requires provision of a respectful and safe space and facilitation that is honest, authentic and non-judgemental. The facilitator must demonstrate compassion and genuine empathy or the group will not develop the trust required for effective participatory action research group work:

'We are very insightful about people's professional acceptance and presence. We need to be believed above all else, so we would only tell someone if we were reasonably confident we might still be accepted and definitely believed. We can tell when someone is disinterested, nosy, perhaps even voyeuristic, judgemental, or labelling us from their textbook reference list instead of listening to our life references. Our life experience has shown us that people often have ulterior motives and hidden agendas when they deal with us. This has made us insightful, even suspicious at times and afraid of people who want to know too many details. We find ourselves asking "How are my details going to help them, and me?" We are worried about not being believed, or being blamed, or judged. Sometimes people do this without realising they do it by asking questions that start with "Why didn't you . . ." and we walk away feeling blamed again, as if we asked for what we got.'

Even though the recall and reflection on the ongoing impact of childhood sexual abuse was painful, one participant revealed a broader agenda as the motivation for her involvement:

'The public do not want to face the fact that child sexual abuse happens. They are too horrified, shocked and stunned and don't know what to do, so they pretend it's not happening in the world that they live in. People in abusive families are ashamed and try to deal with it within the family so they don't lose face or get embarrassed, so the damaging cloak of secrecy continues. We want to diffuse the mystery around this whole dirty subject and help all people see the impact. Our lives have been a living hell and if one good thing comes out of it like these resources from this project then that will at least be something positive for all the pain. We think raising public awareness will help make people confront it, so the perpetrators can find nowhere to hide.'

Facilitating reflection in/on/for action from the 'look-think two step'

Healing from extreme violation such as sexual abuse as a child is a life-long process. The women recognized that the capacity to reflect more clearly was facilitated by guided group work, where they could safely externalize the issue by naming it, and giving it a voice in the group, thus obtaining varying perspectives on the issue. What each woman took from the session, or what changes she instigated in her life was up to her. There were often quite different interpretations for each person:

'Journaling helps me to see I have some good qualities and I find it a healing process. I need to work at finding myself, knowing myself, valuing myself, liking myself, loving myself, and each step is bringing more peace inside myself. I am beginning to like my own company. I enjoy doing my own thing. I am getting stronger by doing things I like, drawing, writing in my journal, doing my workbook and reading books . . .'

It is important that looking and thinking lead to action. Without action, looking and thinking can lead to 'dwelling' and internalization of an issue. Action is like a clearinghouse for issues.

The women found great support in sharing their feelings with people who had travelled the same road, sharing their ways of walking through difficult experiences. Talking was like externalizing the issue and disentangling it from who they were so that they could separate from the abuse. It was like extracting something from inside of them and putting it out into the group to look at. It got issues outside of their heads and into the open space of the group to examine. They were able to hear the perspective of others and see things from different angles. The effectiveness of the group relies on people being willing to put issues into the group space and others being caring.

Looking

In essence the issue/problem/situation was discussed so the woman could make sense of what was happening, increase her understanding, and commence thinking about ways to reshape or re-story her situation. In the safety of the group the story was examined for the woman's meaning first. This could be considered to be what Schön (1983) termed 'reflection-in-action', which takes place when the woman is engaged with her situation and looking and thinking about what is going on, which may produce the tacit knowledge she uses to take further action. The women had a great deal of tacit knowledge about people and survival. Their need to survive their traumatic past had led to highly attuned observation and non-verbal communication skills. Consequently, this group is very able to work out when a health professional is working for/with them as a whole person, or simply focused on their issues. Revealing such tacit knowledge was very useful, because it reinforced the alternate story of survival, resistance, strength and agency, and that story line became the framework for reshaping a new story.

Thinking

Reflection within the participatory action research process is a dynamic movement forwards or backwards. When action does not produce the result intended but rather produces consequences considered to be undesirable, the woman is encouraged to think about why it did not work. Such sense making conversations bring about understandings that can be critiqued, reshaped and embodied, a process that Schön (1983) terms 'reflection-on-action'.

The group provided a safe space for conversations that could be termed 'reflection-for-action', where women considered options, contemplated probable consequences and outcomes of various possible actions, and prioritized their future actions. The outcome was often that the situation took on new meaning, and doing nothing was the chosen action. This was perceived to be an excellent outcome because the woman was choosing to create space to consider the issue before nominating her chosen action.

> 'You do have to talk about it to someone. You have to get it out, because when you are left alone with it you start thinking I can take it, but it just keeps going around and around and digs up all the negative emotions again and you fall back into the hole . . .'

This was an important change from past patterns of responding, which tended to be reactive responses to intense emotions such as fear, anger, guilt and shame.

It was Dewey (1933) who posited reflection as a process that enabled connections to be formed between various aspects of one's experiences. Group reflection facilitated emancipatory knowledge when the women recognized connections between their experiences of abuse, and realised they were not alone in these experiences. Other women had similar thoughts, feelings and emotions that were the legacy of past abuse and this led to a common understanding that helped each woman to feel free to express herself within the group. Interpretive knowledge was facilitated by working together to reflect on their lives, constructing common meanings, making sense of experiences, exploring possible explanations for their current life positions, and thinking through alternative ways of living in the future.

When the women received the previous week's feedback they reflected on the issues discussed. The facilitator thematically clustered common aspects of issues and posed questions that might assist reflective thinking. The narrative conversations shed light on problematic situations that were troubling and uncertain, and enabled each participant to reshape her actions accordingly. First, the issue was named, which could take some time because the women often became confused over the present situation and it took time and patience to establish linkages between current emotions, thoughts, feelings and situations and past experiences. Bearing in mind they had actively suppressed memories, their reflection skills were not a part of their repertoire of life skills. Concurrent with naming things they wished to attend to was framing the context in which they would attend to them (Schön, 1991). The issue was set according to current observations and reflections of experiences. The group compared responses to the framed issue and the women were able to reflect-in-action, coming up with new ways to reframe the initial issue. The group process stimulated reflection, so the women could continue to reframe, experiment, transform knowledge schema and create new insights. With each fortnight a repertoire of life praxis grew and this built a capacity to cope and choose new ways of responding to the intrusions of past sexual abuse on current living and being.

The potential of reflection toward action

The narrative process of group work helped women find solidarity as they worked through their past experiences. There were clusters of common themes that were uncovered in conversations, so new ways of managing the intrusiveness of past trauma could be considered. Particularly intrusive were issues around self-image and self-worth, and emotional experiences such as anger, guilt, shame, fear and anxiety. Horowitz (1976, p. 115) points out that the mind has a 'tendency to seek similarities and integrations'. Consequently, any current experience that provoked such emotional responses within the woman could send her back to former stress responses that she may have chosen to obliterate by using alcohol, drugs or gambling. Over the space of 12 months many of the women could see these connections and understand from where their responses came.

In reflecting about past coping strategies, childhood fantasies and memories, we worked through their life stories, always highlighting any alternate story of strength and resistance. The frequency of the meetings allowed the women to process the issues in manageable bits. They would choose what action to take based on their reflections. Sometimes a woman would absent herself for a time, because she felt the group was causing too many emotional intrusions into her life. Invariably she would use this time to reflect on the therapeutic worth of the group for her current situation. When she was ready she would return. More than 75% of the group chose to return, and are continuing to meet following the conclusion of data generation:

'Before this group my mind sometimes felt like a big wall full of graffiti, but now it's breaking up into clearer pictures.'

The women used their existing repertoire of life-skills and knowledge, reflecting on similarities and differences, to form new understandings and test new propositions within the group, probing their current situation from multiple perspectives:

'The group situation gives me strength and the effects snowball. We talk about real life issues and the positive effect lasts for days for me. It is group problem-solving based on all of our past experiences. We bring our questions and we hear each other's experiences, ideas and different opinions, instead of chasing around with them in our own head.'

Identification of similarities in concepts was described by Schön (1991, p. 183) as developing a generative metaphor that was highlighted in written feedback and became the basis for reflection and the next cycle. These metaphors were used to link ideas, so common ground became obvious, and a sense of solidarity emerged as women could see that they could learn from one another. When they saw that reflection-for-action could lead to significant proactive responses and desired outcomes, they began to see the value in looking, thinking and acting, and began to use this method to solve problems. As with most skills, the more they practised, the better they became at it. Thus the participatory action research process provides participants with emancipatory knowledge and improves their life situation, which is the aim of all participatory action research.

Discussion

The two inquiries discussed in this chapter show the way in which *look*, *think* and *act* may work in a research setting. During the *looking* phase, participants are brought together and given time to become acquainted with each other. Guidelines are developed in consultation with the group. These guidelines for group behaviour create the safety and space for each person to have a voice. Attentive listening and confidentiality are stressed. In the earlier sessions, it is important to explore personal expectations and fears. Participants are often in tune with non-verbal behaviour and can assess the genuineness of the facilitators and others in the group. Participants are invited to tell their own story.

During the *thinking* phase of the group process, disclosure may be a sign that trust has been created; however, it has been noted that trust usually takes several sessions. It took longer for vulnerable client groups, such as the survivors of child sexual abuse, who had inherent difficulty in trusting strangers. There are some revealing character-istics that show that the group is moving, even when there are early signs of anxiety, defensiveness, resistance and a struggle for control. It is recognized that conflict is a part of the group process, which if not addressed can result in defensive behaviour, hostility, indirectness and lack of trust. Effective conflict resolution is likely to result in cohe-sion of the group. The aim of ethical confrontation is to develop a more cohesive and open relationship and it needs to be handled sensitively. It is important to recognize that a person is given an opportunity to reflect before responding to questions raised by others.

In the inquiry with women who were homeless, the movement within one's head of *looking* and *thinking* could quickly become the confusion that triggered panic attacks, anxiety and inability to sleep. Women had multiple health and social issues that could rapidly over-whelm them with fear, anger, guilt, shame, grief, sadness, hopeless-ness and anxiety. These emotions create confusion, and women speak of 'losing their mind' or 'going crazy' (Quas et al., 2003). The women respond to such painful experiences with reactions learned over years of disruption and abuse. As group discussion progressed, it became clear that reacting through taking drugs, alcohol and/or gambling was seen as an immediate response to pain and fear. The fear-driven responses of thinking and reacting (without reflecting) enabled them to survive and provided instant relief. Through expert facilitation, the women learnt to purposefully reflect-on-action and reflect-for-action; it stopped them becoming locked in the dizzying confusion we have termed the 'look-think two step'. Thus, using participatory action research with vulnerable people has the potential to be risky if it is not carefully facilitated.

In the *acting* phase there is usually a commitment of participants to explore issues and there is increased involvement shown by support-ive interactions within the group. Greater responsibility for individual and group outcomes is accepted. Learning is demonstrated by realistic expectations of the group experience. Participants begin to understand that change is often slow and subtle; noticeably, participants make their own decisions regarding what to do with their new knowledge. Often the group's closure includes consolidation of learning and reviewing of experience. When participants are asked what they believe is the most important outcome of the group, they describe the support and recognition they receive from others as being most significant. Often the group continues to meet or converse once the facilitator has left the 'field'. This is most likely to occur if closure is handled sensitively and participants are involved in the closure process.

There are several other characteristics of participatory action research worth declaring:

(1)   It is about building democratic relationships.
(2)   It purposely champions people engaging in its own research.
(3)   People/participants, not researchers, set the agenda for discussion.
(4)   People/participants take control of the entire research process.
(5)   Facilitators (researchers) have special training in researching *with* people.
(6)   Facilitators have an enabling role through strengthening people's awareness of their own capabilities.
(7)   Facilitators create a 'safe' environment for dialogue exchange.
(8)   Participatory action research challenges the traditional science ideal of seeing researchers as neutral and without vested interest; rather, the facilitator's own interests are made apparent (we appeal to reflexivity).
(9)   Knowledge development is a fundamental element in the theory and practice of participatory action research.
(10) Interactions (between individual participants and researchers) are used as data.
(11) Action is facilitated towards human development (individual) and social change (group/community).
(12) The goal of participatory action research is transformation (transition in our research programme may refer to individual and/or group reform).
(13) Findings are constructed and validated collaboratively (participants and researchers).
(14) Research utilization is both a process and product in participatory action research.
(15) Cooperation between participants and researchers supports significant change processes.
(16) Cooperation between participants and researchers creates a context for bringing forth new theory connected to the deepest challenges of change.

Summary

These characteristics reflect our participatory action research practice as it has evolved over the last decade of collaborative inquiries. We celebrate the diversity of sources that have inspired us. No doubt our participatory action research approach will increase in sophistication as we continue to research with participants and continue to learn.

10 Rigour and Quality

This chapter's aim is to stimulate debate about rigour and quality in participatory action research. There is a vast literature surrounding rigour concerned with 'rule governed approaches' and we do not wish to add to these rules. However, it is important to consider ways in which participatory action research may be seen as a rigorous approach. At the same time it seems important to ask whether participatory action research work is accessible, makes a difference and is sustainable. These are questions about quality. We argue that rigour and quality of participatory action research practice are co-dependent. In this chapter, guidelines for reading participatory action research inquiries are offered. Our observations of rigour are based on our experiences in researching alongside participants during the last decade.

Reading for rigour

Whilst participants have the final say in making the decision about an inquiry's quality, we practice action research in a world in which we are expected to demonstrate rigour. The stakes are high when deciding whether a research inquiry using participatory action research is believable, plausible and/or trustworthy. Arguing for the legitimacy of participatory action research approaches may not concern participants as much as those who fund participatory action research inquiries. If rigour and/or quality claims are dismissed we may not have access to funding for subsequent years. It is important that those working in the field are cognisant of the debates surrounding participatory action research and that action researchers understand ways they can argue for participatory action research as a legitimate endeavour. We hope to alert you to some of the strategies that may be useful in participatory action research and consider ways in which 'rigour' claims can be made when 'findings' are presented.

A review of literature on rigour shows that researchers during the 1980s struggled to apply criteria used in quantitative research to qualitative work (Koch & Harrington, 1998). Then in the late 1980s researchers adapted the parallel criteria of credibility, transferability and dependability for the assessment of qualitative work. Guided by the work of Guba & Lincoln (1989), Koch (1994, 1998) and Koch & Harrington (1998), here are some questions regarding rigour worth considering.

- What is the world view?
- Is the inquiry credible?
- Is the inquiry transferable?
- Is the study dependable?
- Is the study believable?
- What are the values and interests researchers bring to the inquiry?
- Is the work accessible?

What is the author's world view? In the introduction we have argued that our version of participatory action research has emerged from our world view, which we identified as a participative world view. This world view drives participatory action research processes. Consistent with this world view is that participatory action research is motivated by a desire to secure authentic information about people and situations studied that is useful for stakeholders in health care delivery, particularly clients and community. Although not always feasible, the main aim is to involve participants in every phase of the research process. In order to make quality assessments, participants validate findings in cycles of reflection and action. Participation in the entire process promises that the findings are relevant, believable and useful. Participant ownership of the research inquiry may sustain action processes into the future. Outcomes, in terms of human flourishing, continue to impact on the lives of those involved in the inquiry. Whenever we write we aim to draw the reader's attention to participative world view aspects of our participatory action research inquiries. When you read participatory action research work, question what the author's world view is.

Is the inquiry credible? It is important to show that people's voices are represented adequately. 'The metaphor of voice is common to feminist and action research' (Maguire, 2001, p. 63). Drawing from Freire's (1970) work to pierce the culture of silence among marginalized groups, participatory research is fundamentally about the right to speak (Maguire, 2001). One way in which we have engaged our participants is by writing stories that are meaningful and make sense in their own lives. Telling a vital story about the inquiry provides context and information. It captures the mood of the setting and presents voices that make the experience come alive. Even though we are guided by the ethical guideline of anonymity, participants recognize their own voice and this assures them they have been heard. When reading participatory action research text, participants often say that 'it is right, that it is interesting, that it is engaging or that it is thought provoking' (Bradbury & Reason, 2001, p. 449). Participants are part of the entire validation process and a reader may seek evidence to support this claim. Consensus may not be the outcome but if differences and divergences are observed, it is important to show how interpretations were derived from data generated. An inquiry may be considered credible when multiple voices are heard in inquiry reports. It is credible when co-researchers (our participants) as key producers and consumers of the inquiry report, view the findings as meaningful and relevant in their lives. Can readers trace interpretations and show they are firmly grounded in the data?

Is the inquiry transferable? Using the criterion of transferability, which may allow us to transfer findings from one research inquiry to another, consider the similarities. This requires the researcher to describe the context, not only the setting but also a profile of the participants. The original context must be described adequately so that a judgement of transferability can be made. Of course, resultant group actions or reforms a group has instigated are not transferable but sometimes the theoretical notions arising from an inquiry can be transferred. Our inquiries with people living with chronic illness have shown that the emerging transition thesis is supported by individual inquiries. That is to say, findings are transferable. If we commence a group with a description of transition previously validated by a participatory action research group, we can often continue to build on this understanding. We would not start from scratch with every group; rather, we share our current research and ask participants whether transition concepts can be transferred into their lives; in so doing we continue to build our construction collaboratively. The profiles of participants, the people who live with a variety of chronic conditions, provide the context. However, whilst all have chronic conditions, our participants are predominantly middle class, have reached a reasonable educational standard and often have access to computers. Already gender differences have shifted our understandings of transition and it would not surprise us if class, race and ethnicity were to shape alternative understandings. If transferability of context is intimately tied to participant profiles, are these given?

Is the study dependable? One of the ways in which a research study may be shown to be dependable is for its process to be audited. An inquiry audit of this type is based on the fiscal audit undertaken to authenticate the accounts of a business. In the same way that the auditor examines the process by which accounts are kept in order to exclude the possibility of error or fraud, the decision trail can be established as a means for the researcher to provide audit trail linkages. This is what is meant by dependability. Systematic research processes are hall marks of any rigorous research, and the point here is maintaining a record of methodological decisions, e.g. how data are generated, analysed and described, is one aspect of that record. All decisions and choices made whilst researching are made visible in the text. Theoretical, methodological and analytical choices can provide a framework for recording and analysing a decision trail. Has the author considered ways in which the inquiry may be dependable?

Is the study believable? Reflexivity provides answers to Gadamer's (1976) question: 'What is going on in methods?' Gadamer does not provide us with a method, he suggests we record and analyse what is going on whilst we are researching, thus providing a context for our decisions as we move through the process of research. Monitoring 'what is going on' requires that reflexivity is maintained throughout the research process. We are already engaged in cycles of reflection and action with participants, but alongside this we need to record what is going on whilst engaged in the participatory action research process. This means considering the entire research process as a reflexive exercise. Through making the entire research process visible a reader can make a decision about the inquiry's plausibility, believability or trustworthiness. Is the reader able to follow the signposts and grasp 'what is going on' while researching?

What are the values and interests researchers bring to the inquiry? We contend that researchers bring data generated, a range of literature, a positioning of this literature, a positioning of oneself, and moral socio-political contexts. In addition to taking account of the author's world view, researchers' interests influence the way in which a research inquiry develops. It is a reminder to record and analyse influences, at least those accessible to us, whilst researching. This reflexive account is characterized by ongoing self-critique and self-appraisal and by the fact that the research product can be given shape by the politics of location and positioning. Maintaining a daily journal and analysing the contents is the strategy here. Are values and interests declared and does subsequent writing incorporate a reflexive account into the inquiry report?

Is the work accessible? One of the most startling characteristics of participatory action research is ongoing validation of data, stories and analysis. The most desirable end product is the text that has been co-constructed. Although the text is co-constructed, it is the researcher's responsibility to bring all aspects of the work together. When possible, participants assist with writing, but mostly they are critical consumers of the researcher's written work. Nevertheless, participants have access to all writings arising from the inquiry. Cycles of feedback are part of the process. The work should be engaging, otherwise few people will read it. People living with chronic conditions and clinicians have officially joined us in publication and this is a highly desirable outcome. Clinician involvement is evidenced by clinicians acting as co-authors on papers and presenting research findings at conferences. Where possible, we facilitate clinician involvement at every aspect of the research process; however organizational and workload constraints have sometimes prevented this. One way to make findings accessible is to disseminate these throughout key organizations and tertiary institutions in a monthly newsletter, which is posted on the Internet. It is vital that written accounts are accessible. In which ways has the inquiry report been made accessible?

How are we to evaluate a participatory action research study? Is the interpretation convincing? Is the inquiry rigorous? We claim that if the inquiry is well signposted the readers will be able to decide for themselves whether the text is trustworthy, believable or plausible.

Questions about quality

Is the inquiry useful? Has it made a difference and are actions sustained? How do we know we have a quality research practice? Involvement of all stakeholders in cyclical processes means we learn and record whether the inquiry is useful, has made a difference and whether actions can be sustained.

Recently, action researchers have merged rigour and quality debates. The most influential ideas are drawn from Reason & Bradbury (2001) who ask 'Am I doing good work?' Their concern, like ours, is not about advancing rule-governed approaches but about extending a useful conversation about getting valuable work done well. An appealing description of their approach is that 'research is best seen as an emergent, evolutionary and educational process of engaging with self, persons, and communities which needs to be sustained for a significant period of time' (Reason & Bradbury, 2001, p. 11). These authors use the term validity, not rigour. We discuss their work next.

Characteristics of action research have been identified and this has led these authors to ask five kinds of questions about the validity and quality of action research practice. These are taken from the final chapter in the *Handbook of Action Research* (Reason & Bradbury, 2001, p. 454).

Questions for quality in action research

Is action research:

(1) Explicit in developing praxis of relational participation?
(2) Guided by reflexive concern for practical outcomes?

(3) Inclusive of a plurality of knowing?
Ensuring conceptual-theoretical integrity?
Embracing ways of knowing beyond the intellect?
Intentionally choosing appropriate research methods?
(4) Worthy of the term significant?
(5) Emerging towards a new and enduring infrastructure?

The authors give these questions as 'choice points'. That is, an action research inquiry may not be able to address all of these questions, but researchers may have considered some of these questions that relate to their practice. In return these questions may stimulate discussion and help us to make decisions about the quality of action research practice.

Questions about relational practice

Building relationships is a pivotal experience when researching with people. More importantly, 'action research emerges from a participative way of seeing the world in which we find ourselves always in relationships' (Bradbury & Reason, 2001, p. 448). Our interpretation of relationships is tied to responsibilities as researchers in paying attention to the creation of safe environments for dialogue, honing our awareness of group dynamics, observing and monitoring power relations, and facilitating growth and development; in short, we prioritize building an environment where relationships can thrive. Often relationships continue once we have left the field. Most often, in the evaluation of the participatory action research process, participants describe the impact others have had on their learning experiences. The relationship dimension draws our attention to the quality of the interaction that has been developed in the inquiry and the political forms that have been developed to sustain the inquiry. Bradbury and Reason ask:

- How have the values of democracy been actualized in practice?
- What is the relationship between initiator and participants?
- What are the implications for infrastructure and political structures?

Our research practice has been guided by Ernie Stringer's work (Box 10.1).
Again these are useful principles when considering participatory action research and when reading participatory action research text. A record of some of these principles may be incorporated into the inquiry report.

Box 10.1 Working principles of community based action research.

Relationships in action research:
- Promote feelings of equality for all people involved
- Maintain harmony
- Avoid conflicts where possible
- Resolve conflicts that arise, openly and dialogically
- Accept people as they are, not as some people think they ought to be
- Encourage personal, cooperative relationships, rather than impersonal, competitive, conflicting or authoritarian relationships
- Be sensitive to people's needs

In effective communication:
- Listen attentively to people
- Accept and act upon what is said
- Ensure the conversation can be understood by everyone
- Be truthful and sincere
- Act in socially and culturally appropriate ways
- Regularly advise others about what is happening

Participation is most effective when it:
- Enables significant levels of active involvement
- Enables people to perform significant tasks
- Provides support for people as they learn and act for themselves
- Encourages plans and activities that people are able to accomplish themselves
- Deals personally with people rather than with their representatives or agents

Inclusion in action research involves:
- Maximization of the involvement of all relevant individuals
- Inclusion of all relevant issues – (social, economic, cultural, political), rather than focusing on a narrow administrative or political agendas
- Ensures cooperation with other groups, agencies and organizations
- Ensures that relevant groups benefit from activities

(Stringer, 1999, p. 38)

Questions of outcomes and practice

As we were writing this section, an email message arrived from a woman with whom we have been researching for 2 years. Here are her responses to our evaluation questions:

What has been your experience of being involved in the group?
An incredible relief to be able to talk about how I feel physically without the stigma of being told others are not interested, etc. To have someone have a clue how you feel with chronic fatigue has been so helpful.

What has it been like to share your experiences in the group?
Freeing, helpful to find and follow up links.

What discussions were most helpful?
I think all have been helpful, but I have a feeling I missed out on a couple of questions.

What discussions weren't helpful?
None.

What did you learn?
The reaffirmation that you are not alone, that there are always those who are worse off, but that there is a community in pain, etc., as there is in other life experiences.

What surprised you?
I could be honest about how I felt . . . just no energy, etc., and not be judged.

What has changed for you since being involved in the group?
I am probably more isolated and have retreated more and bore my friends less with how I am now that I am part of an email group.

What didn't you like about being involved in the group?
Nothing annoyed me too much.

What did you like best about being involved in the group?
Sharing, caring, and standing together.

Although these questions were posted only 2 hours earlier, her quick spontaneous response indicates that without doubt the participatory action research group has been significant in this person's life. She feels empowered, less stigmatized and being part of the group has made a difference. This person has said the work was useful and she is using what she has learned. Fortunately this woman's group will continue once the inquiry has ceased.

Reason & Bradbury (2001, p. 11) ask:

* What are the outcomes of the research?
* Does it work?
* What are the processes of inquiry?
* Are they authentic/life enhancing?

Another way outcomes can be assessed is by asking pragmatic questions about the inquiry. Here we strive to be reflexive about our practice and respond to the question 'What is going on whilst researching?'

As stated earlier, it is important to us that the work we do is meaningful and has the potential to make a difference. Kemmis (2001)
reminds us that outcomes can be expressed in technical, practical
and/or emancipatory terms and these distinctions (from Habermas) are
quite useful. It seems that the longer we are in contact with our participants, the more likely those outcomes will cross the three categories.

When we first commence working alongside participatory action
research participants, outcomes tend to be technical and practical.
Take the tentative beginning when working with older people living
with asthma, who in the first weeks of the inquiry, voiced that they
were hungry for medical information (Koch et al., 2003). They asked
for current medication management information, and as they set the
agenda, this was provided at the level requested. Subsequently there
were improved self-management outcomes to report. This mode of
inquiry is a single loop inquiry, 'seeking merely to get things accomplished' (Reason & Bradbury, 2001, p. 448). Moving towards a double
loop inquiry, we must then ask about the value of the things we have
accomplished. When participants have been researching alongside us
for a while, the reflection/action cycle stimulates their thinking
beyond immediate technical/practical outcomes.

In the effort to explain a double loop or emancipatory outcome we
might say that the major constraint to asthma self-management was its
narrow conception as solely medical management. Those participants with
asthma since childhood were experts in their own self-management,
although not always acknowledged as such. They were expert about
their own lives. Here the term 'self-management' refers to the activities
these people have undertaken to create order, discipline and control in
their lives. Whilst earlier outcomes show that improved self-management
of medication is highly regarded in the medicalized world, outcomes
from a second loop or another level draw attention to the shift from
medical self-management to authentic self-management. Participants,
although clearly in charge of managing themselves, were for the first
time being acknowledged as proficient managers of their asthma.
Participatory action research group validation was empowering for
participants. It offered them another way of seeing themselves and they
liked their new identities. So in the same inquiry, there was scope for
single and double loop outcomes. Participants were conversant with
medical asthma management in the first instance and managed the 'self'
in the context of their lives in the second.

Questions about ways of knowing

'Each particular way of knowing raises questions concerning quality
in its own right' (Bradbury & Reason 2001, p. 448). Referring to the inquiry

with people living with asthma, the first claim, of improved self-medication management, is seen as a legitimate outcome by medical management practitioners. The second claim, inferring that individuals have expert knowledge to manage illness in their own lives, is not considered to be a legitimate knowledge claim by those same practitioners. The questions about ways of knowing we could ask are:

- How well is an inquiry experientially grounded?
- Does it promote further knowing by allowing us to see 'through' old conceptual frameworks?
- Is the new way of seeing enabling or limiting?

As readers we could ask:

- What is the appropriate form of presentation given the audience?
- Is it aesthetically elegant?
- Is it conceptually clear to all involved?

Reflection on ways of knowing encourages us to ask what dimensions of an extended epistemology are emphasized in the inquiry and whether this is appropriate. It encourages us to consider the validity of the claims of the different forms of knowing and the relationships between different ways of knowing (Reason & Bradbury, 2001, p. 11). These are questions about plural ways of knowing.

The choice and rationale for selection of approach are closely related to the quality of the inquiry. We use among other data generation strategies, interviews, participatory action research groups and email correspondence, and make a claim that these inquiries are congruent with our participative world view. 'Participatory research is an attitude, a way of creating knowing in action' (Reason & Bradbury, 2001, p. 449).

Questions about purpose and significance

Three questions are about the work we do. Is it important? Is it is worthwhile? What values have been actualized in the inquiry? Two of these questions can be answered by participants, the third is the outcome of ongoing reflections of both researchers and participants.

Emergent theories as a result of sequential inquiries tend to persuade external funding bodies that there is significant progress in theory building. Chapter 11 will show theory development across inquiries; here we will use an example from practice and walk the reader through a theory building process within one inquiry.

Transition theory is the product of a collaborative process *with* participants

Exploring transition with people who live with a chronic illness is part of a 3 year longitudinal inquiry. We invite people to talk, and in so doing, they share experiences that provide focus and context about living with a chronic condition. Over time, experiences shared begin to resemble life stories. With participants as the central characters of their stories, we witness shifts in self-identity. Collaboratively we gather, analyse and reshape stories.

When we trace both individual and group stories, common assumptions about people living with chronic illness are disputed or contested. Theorizing *with* participants has meant showing that what we take for granted has been historically constructed. This theory provides a confrontational critique of common sense notions and a challenge to biomedical constructions of illness. Whilst the transition theory is certainly a critique of common sense notions it is also an exploration of alternative constructions. Alternative constructions offer ways in which people, research participants, significant others and health care professionals, can think differently about living with a chronic illness.

What is a story?

The shape, ebb and form of the story are results of ongoing consultation and negotiation. A transition story is about the past, present and the future. The past is the most suitable context and genre for self-making. Prioritizing participants' voices while simultaneously recognizing the impact of the researcher is a key concern. In the effort to co-construct stories, individual stories are traced, brought together by the facilitator, returned to the participants, and revised and rewritten collaboratively. In the creation of stories, alternate interpretations are important. Their articulation is crucial to the emancipation process. The way in which the writer deals with atypical encounters/stories is important. From these individual stories a larger 'common' transition story is woven.

What is the process?

Active telling occurs in conjunction with others. The shaping of the story, the analysis of the narration and its editing are done in collaboration *with* participants. Reflexivity of the researchers is paramount and these accounts are woven into the product. Focus on the role of the researcher/facilitator is maintained at all stages of the research process. This asks for a transparent approach to positioning the researcher in relation to the emancipatory frame, where writers' political and theoretical orientations are revealed openly throughout the process.

Steering of the research can be monitored through revelations delivered by facilitator.

What is meant by with?

Transparency about the process means talking with others in terms of dialogue and interpretation. Dialogue allows the meanings of self in relation to others to be communicated. So the story being told relies on active engagement with the participants. Whilst the writer has the final authority regarding the story of transition, the process is guided and shaped by the men and women with whom we research.

Who are the participants and where are their voices?

The emancipatory framework from this account:

- allows joint ownership of the story of transition;
- acknowledges the gains made by the researcher from the generation of data;
- provides a process rather than presuming that analysis can enlighten the story teller;
- means doing research ethically so that participants might usefully gain something from the process and production; and
- leads to the story arising from sustained collaboration and negotiation between researchers and participants.

Analysis

What are the common assumptions about people living with chronic illness? What are the common sense notions? What is disputed or contested? What are biomedical constructions of illness? What are alternative constructions?

Thinking about reflexivity has elucidated two aspects of the research process: the nature of the research relationship and its relationship to ontology, epistemology and methodology in theory construction. The research relationship is personified in analysis through engagement with participants in constant conversation cycles. This ensures that the analyst attends to the meaning held by participants. Stories are woven together by the facilitator for both individuals and the groups.

Questions about enduring consequence

Is the work sustainable into the future? The most important relationships are not those we forge through the participatory action research process but those remaining once we have left. When relationships thrive, resultant individual and group action is likely to be sustained. Participatory action research, as an orientation to reform, change and transition, is exceptional as a research approach. Individuals, groups and community can and do move forward as they embrace another way of viewing the world. We talk about closure as if it happens. In reality, participants continue to converse with us, as friends, long after the inquiry has ceased. These informal conversations support our claim that many actions are sustained, but formal evaluations are required. Rather than rely on anecdote, these evaluations need to take place 1 to 2 years after the inquiry has been completed. However, evaluation of enduring consequences is often on hold while we explore opportunities for further funding. Rarely are external grants available allowing us to return to the inquiry several years later to assess it effects. A stronger argument needs to be formulated for funding that allows researchers to meet with participants several years later to ask the pertinent question 'What has changed?'

Summary

In this chapter we ask the reader of an inquiry report to consider rigour by asking the questions: What is the world view? Is the inquiry credible? Is the inquiry transferable? Is the study dependable? Is the study believable? What are the values and interests that researchers bring to the inquiry? Is the work accessible? We have included Stringer's (1999) principles, which may guide inquiry.

Five choice points are given for asking quality questions. Relationships, practice outcomes, extended ways of knowing, purpose and enduring consequence, are choice points from the Reason & Bradbury (2001) handbook. Expectations would be frustrated if we were to incorporate all aspects into an inquiry. Rather they are choice points and each researcher is able to consider which they may prefer or what is feasible within one inquiry. Questions raised in this chapter will hopefully alert action researchers to consider rigour and quality issues in their work, writing and research outcomes.

11 Transition and Theory Building

Co-authored by Dr Anne van Loon

When undertaking a review of action research literature in the effort to identify themes and trends, Dick (2004) proposed that theory development is scarce in this field and he questioned the reasons for its absence. In this chapter we offer a developing theory of transition. We have clearly articulated our aim to make a difference in health care and we believe that theory is defined by its practical relevance. Theories are after all, words on paper that can only offer guidance about phenomena. The meaning occurs in practice. Theories stimulate thinking and offer a springboard for further knowledge development, which is our intent in sharing this developing work.

A decade of systematic inquiry with people who live with a chronic illness has enabled us to build an understanding of 'transition'. We define transition as the way in which people have learnt to absorb the consequences of living through a disruptive life event such as chronic illness and then create a sense of continuity again. This process has been the centre of theoretical development. Building theory collaboratively with community dwelling participants has been the distinguishing feature of our research programme and approach to participatory action research.

Theory development

In each of the inquiries we have undertaken we have explored with people, common assumptions about their experiences of living with chronic illness. In so doing we have been challenged to question the assumptions about the experience of chronic illness that we have developed over decades as health workers. We have realized that theory creation is often a confrontational critique of common sense notions and a challenge to biomedical constructions of illness. Theorizing means attempting to show that what we take for granted has been historically constructed. Theory is insightful when it surprises and challenges, when it encourages us to imaginatively see phenomena that we thought we had understood. Whilst it is a critique of common sense it is also an exploration of alternative constructions. In order to make a difference, we need to show what our theory disputes. The theory must offer ways in which people, research participants, significant others and health care professionals, can think differently about living with chronic illness. The effect we desire through theorizing is to shift people's views. The presentation of the developing transition theory can be considered as a stepping stone for future rigorous theoretical investigations questioning 'when, how, and why'. Guided by participants, reshaping our practice to listen, learn and understand is the core of the reform we envisage.

Why have we utilized participatory action research processes? Over the past decade the language of participation has become increasingly prevalent within health care practice and systems. Underpinning the principle of participation is the idea that community ownership and empowerment are crucial in supporting and effecting change. There is growing recognition within the health care industry and government that the vision of social, ecological and economic sustainability depends on building social capacity, as well as economic and physical resources. This is particularly evident around the area of chronic illness, with a focus towards self-care or self-management (Redman, 2004). The processes of participatory action research fit well within this context.

The cyclical nature of the participatory action research process promotes reflection and reconstruction of experiences and story that can lead to the enhancement of people's lives, at an individual level, community level, or both. As discussed earlier, our involvement in participatory action research inquiries with people who live with a chronic illness has enabled us to build theory from participatory action research. Building theory collaboratively with community dwelling participants has been a distinguishing feature of our research programme.

We have worked towards consolidating the findings from our chronic illness research programme and moved towards theory development by continually revising and validating the emerging constructs evolving from the stories of participants. The transition theory provides a continuum of chronic illness experience, and demonstrates patterns among and between data from multiple inquiries. In addition, our analysis and interpretation has occurred and reshaped over time as we have undertaken longitudinal studies with people who are living through disruption. Our reason has been to understand the movement people experience, the way their perceptions and actions change over time, which is fundamental to the transition process.

Our focus has been to determine the experience of transition as movement 'through' disruption, which implies a process of change, rather than a 'from-to', which suggests there are often discrete starting and ending points of transition (Saldana, 2003). On the contrary, we have found that transition is fluid, often convoluted movement occurring throughout our lives.

Before we introduce our theoretical understanding of transition, we should acknowledge that this is an introduction to theory development arising from participatory action research. It is beyond the scope of this chapter to give but a summary glance at the work we are accomplishing. A full discussion of transition will be material for another book.

Transition

When people are living with chronic illness, it is paramount to learn and develop the capacity to adapt in a world of challenge and transition (Redman, 2004). A chronic illness is one that persists over time, usually without an easily definable beginning, middle or end (Kralik, 2002). While the symptoms of chronic illness may be alleviated to some extent, the illness itself is not curable.

The transition theory exposes a process of learning to adapt to life's adverse disruptions, such as chronic illness, by utilizing processes inherent in participatory action research that may strengthen a person's capacity to move through the disruption towards a sense of living well. We have chosen to explain the transition process in a linear fashion; however, the phenomena we are explaining do not occur in linear order. Transition is a messy life process! In our description of transition we attempt to show what is experienced by our participants, connect these understandings to current literature, and create cycles of reflection and action. Our intention has been to understand and describe the process of transition. The description we offer is in collaboration with many participants. We will share ways in which health workers may intervene to assist people through the transitional processes.

Literature

Theoretical development and reviews of literatures are ongoing. As sophistication increases, the construct of transition is always on the move as we incorporate new understandings. In current literature, the meaning of transition has varied with the context in which the term has been used. Transition has evolved in the social sciences and health disciplines, with nurses contributing to more recent understandings of the transition process as it relates to life and health (Chick & Meleis, 1986; Cantanzaro, 1990; Loveys, 1990; Meleis & Trangenstein, 1994; Schumacher & Meleis, 1994; Meleis et al., 2000; Kralik, 2002).

Definitions of transition are shaped by disciplinary focus, but most agree transition involves a passage of change. A common definition of transition cited within health disciplines is:

> 'A passage from one life phase, condition, or status to another . . . transition refers to both the process and the outcome of complex person-environment interactions. It may involve more than one person and is embedded in the context and the situation. Defining characteristics of transition include process, disconnectedness perception and patterns and response.'
> (Chick & Meleis, 1986, pp. 239–240)

A concept analysis was presented by Meleis et al. (2000) that provided both a perspective and a framework for understanding transitions such as developmental, health, socio-cultural, situational, relational and organisational changes and critical events. It was proposed that people may undergo more than one transition at any given time and that it is important for the person to be aware of the changes taking place and engage with them (Meleis et al., 2000). Possible indicators that transition is occurring included:

- the individual feels connected to, and interacts with, his/her situation and other people;
- the individual feels located or situated so that he/she can reflect and interact; and
- the individual develops increased confidence in coping with changes and mastering new skills and ways of living, while developing a more flexible sense of identity in the midst of changes (Meleis et al., 2000).

Transition occurs when a person's current reality is disrupted, causing a forced or chosen change that results in the need to construct a new reality (Selder, 1989). Transition can only occur if the person is aware of the changes that are taking place (Chick & Meleis, 1986). This awareness is then followed by engagement, where one is immersed in the transition process and undertakes activities such as seeking information or support, identifying new ways of living and being, modifying former activities, and making sense of circumstances. Therefore one's level of awareness will influence one's level of engagement, with lack of awareness signifying an individual may not be ready for transition (Meleis et al., 2000). Both Bridges (1980, 2004) and Selder (1989) highlighted the importance of personal acknowledgment that a prior way of living/being has ended, or a current reality is under threat and that change needs to occur before the transition process can begin. Once this acknowledgment occurs one can begin to make sense of what is happening and reorganize a new way to live, respond and be in the world. The process of surfacing awareness involves noticing what has changed and how things are different (Meleis et al., 2000; Kralik, 2002). Dimensions of difference that can be explored include the nature of the changes, how long they are likely to occur, what possible trajectory they may follow, the perceived importance and severity of changes, and the personal, familial and societal influences impacting on the changes (Meleis et al., 2002). Kralik (2002) noted that people in transition feel different, may be perceived by others as different, and that they view their world in a different way, as a result of the movement that occurs during transition. We contend that transition is about moving through the disruption caused by difference.

Transition is not just another word for change (Bridges, 2004), but rather the psychological processes involved in adapting to the change event or disruption. Transition is the movement and adaptation to change, rather than a return to a pre-existing state. Bridges (2004, p. 11) stated 'every transition begins with an ending', meaning that people have to let go of the familiar ways of being in the world that defined who they were. This is particularly important for health professionals, who are most often supporting people through forced disruptions such as illness (Kralik, 2002). Transitional processes require time as people gradually disengage from old habits and behaviours and ways of defining self. This represents a profound departure from the medical model of problematizing illness and change, to health professionals working alongside people to identify new possibilities. We do not argue that the biomedical discourse is inappropriate or should be replaced; on the contrary we accept that biomedical discourses focus on achieving specific outcomes, but argue that the biomedical discourse does not allow acknowledgement of this sense of transition. Understanding transitions offers a framework that will enable health professionals to move beyond the biomedically orientated concepts of health practice, towards a holistic approach to the provision of care (Kralik, 2002).

Health professionals can work with people who are in the midst of profound disruption by listening to their stories, sensitively acknowledging the issues and conflicts identified, and collaboratively planning action to address issues. This type of positive, respectful interaction conveys a strong message to the individual that he or she is a valued human being and contributes to the reconstruction of a valued self-identity that has been identified as essential to transition.

Developing theory of transition

Transition is about moving through disruption to a place where continuity again takes precedence. Social or cultural expectations, meanings and roles structure our lives. Disruption inevitably occurs as it interrupts or ends our familiar lives, the daily order of our lives, and a degree of predictability that we take for granted. When expectations about the course of life are not met or seem threatened, people experience disruption. Disruption is about difference and represents a perceived change in future. 'Restoring some order to life necessitates reworking understandings of the self and the world, redefining the disruption and life itself' (Becker, 1997, p. 4). Restoring continuity or order, guided by the experiences of our participants, seems to be a human need. Stories of transition engage issues of power, starting with language such as victimization, disconnection and uncertainty. Describing the process of transitional movement, our language shifts to terms such as mastery and resilience, in the effort to reclaim order in life. People's initial focus following a disruptive event or experience is about loss of control over their lives. Whether the disruption has caused a lifetime of powerlessness, such as women who were sexually violated during childhood, or has been a more recent impact, such as adult onset chronic illness, the imbalance of power is experienced through constructs of normalizing according to cultural and societal norms. This is what we mean by stories of disruption being essentially stories of difference. The theory of transition is about creating order from disruption.

In the process of creating order from disruption, a pathway has been identified. As discussed earlier, whilst our presentation is linear, transition is a messy business and it certainly does not follow a straight pathway. However, for the purpose of description, we have identified several constructs: familiar life, ending, limbo and becoming ordinary. We will discuss these constructs more closely.

Familiar life

Most of us have experienced the comfort, stability, security and contentment that our familiar lives bring. The familiar is not only about our past but is also about our present and the illusion and skewed perspective of certainty we have of what the future holds. The ordinary is captured in the repetitiveness of our lives. Our identities relate to our social roles as mother, father, daughter, son, partner, academic, teacher, nurse, etc. A sense of self alludes to who we are, where we are, and where we are going. This gives the person a sense of order, integrity and inner peace that promotes health and self-esteem and fosters self-identity.

Everyday life can be so familiar and routine that we often fail to see and experience what is happening around us. We wake up, prepare for our day, travel the same roads to work, do our jobs thinking very little about what could be different, and at the end of the day we return to the sameness of each evening. There exists a sense of safety through continuity, of life as being ordinary and flowing. We know that there are places and routines and ways of relating and being with one another that we can count on and trust. It is only when something goes wrong that we reflect.

Ending

Every experience of transition begins with an ending. The disruptive event ends the sense of continuity, order and the familiar. Throughout our lives, people deal constantly with endings and we go through the process without much thought at all. However, some endings trouble us greatly. People may be fearful of the change and the unknown, and desperately yearn for the familiar and the comfortable.

The disruptive event is usually unexpected or forced, meaning that people have had little, if any choice of the event occurring. The ending represents the immediate aftermath of change. People have ideals about order and normalcy. Depending on the nature of the disrupting event, they may be challenged by various cultural ideals, for example of health and illness, being a woman or a man, or being a parent. People may come into conflict with the social order as they perceive it. For example, if illness is the disrupting event, the individual may have a sense of being damaged and have a fear of change, and disconnection to the familiar. Disruption and difference pervade, bringing with them feelings of vulnerability.

In western culture our life search is about our pursuit of meaning, purpose, order, integrity and inner peace, aiming to avoid disruption and disorientation. We are confronted when an event or situation disrupts our status quo and forces us to end one way of living that may have achieved these goals. People then attempt to make sense of what has ended and often re-invent their sense of self in the midst of these changes. Through incorporating changed circumstances into their lives, people are enabled to regain a sense of meaning and purpose, thus re-establishing the sense of identity. This sounds straightforward enough, except that there are many instances where the options for change are unclear, choices are reduced and the personal capacity to reflect and act is limited.

Limbo

A state of limbo occurs between previous identities and the new. It is a time when the old way is gone and the new way of thinking about oneself does not feel comfortable. There is an overwhelming sense of being different, which compounds feelings of isolation, vulnerability, loss, guilt and dependency.

Limbo is the murky area between the old and the new, where people struggle to let go of the past and realign themselves with a shift in identity, and new goals and aspirations. There can be an overwhelming sense of loss and people can see what had been forgone but are yet to see what possibilities lie before them. People may dwell with their feelings and self-absorption often predominates as they begin working through the transitional processes. This period of self-absorption may alienate people from others. It can be a period of confusion and emptiness in which the person locates what has ended. Many people need to withdraw for a period of time to do the self-examination and introspection required to make sense of what is happening, so they can work out how it has affected their sense of identity.

Preoccupation with disruption appears to be unavoidable, but in its wake, it fosters learning. Learning encourages adjusting the way we live. It seems we need to reflect our feelings and experience a moratorium from the conventional activity of our everyday existences (Bridges, 2004). The inner shift, the transition, does not happen as quickly as the outer shift, the change. The familiar is gone, but the new beginning is not obvious yet.

Being in limbo may be a time that is marked by activity. Conversely, this may also be an empty time in which not much seems to be happening. The future is not clear but the past is gone. The past may not be gone in a literal sense because the same people may still be around, many of the surroundings and support systems may be in place. Yet people feel that their lives are unanchored.

This is a difficult period for people who like clarity and definition in their lives. In response to the uncertainty, people try to put the new in place as quickly as possible, even though they may not be ready. Time and space is needed to assist people to understand what can be done, what should be done, why people feel the way they do, and what people need. Mourning the loss of the old, as we struggle to grasp hold of the new, we conjure up a limbo, within which we can begin to build a foundation for what is to come. Paradigm shifts leave people feeling confused as customary life patterns are slowly being replaced by new ideas and actions.

Becoming ordinary

Becoming ordinary is the process of new beginnings. The confusion and disruption begin to give way to new possibilities that are devised and revised. Events, perceptions and identity begin to reshape and life begins to take focus. Becoming ordinary creates a new identity and involves reconstructing and revising life whilst coming to terms with the new in the light of actually living the new. It is an ongoing process, which redefines itself over and over again, until it no longer is a beginning. Becoming ordinary involves letting go and saying goodbye to the familiar so that change may occur. By learning how to end things, people learn how to begin things; however, it takes time to integrate changes into daily life.

People acknowledge that a prior way of living/being has ended, or a current reality is under threat and that change needs to occur

Box 11.1 Transition – a process of convoluted passage during which people redefine their sense of self and redevelop self-agency in response to disruptive life events.

Familiar life	Ending	Limbo	Becoming ordinary
Living and being in the world is predictable and situations are taken for granted.	The current way of living ends. The change event or experience may be chosen or forced but life is different.	The changes, chosen or forced, may become disorientating. It can be a time of suffering and disempowerment. Moving through this phase is facilitated by sense-making activities.	Incorporating changing patterns of being and doing into new ways of living. Living life in a way that provides a sense of coherence.
In our familiar lives we experience: • predictability • identity • roles • status • location • situation • security • relationships • connections • acquaintances • internalized socio-cultural norms • thoughts feelings attitudes within self • ordinary life	Following an ending we may experience: • disruption • difference • fractured identity • brokenness • being over burdened • fear • displacement • separation • disconnection • uncertainty • hesitation • insecurity • ambiguity • vulnerability • inadequacy • violation • victimization	During limbo we may experience: • confusion • turmoil • uncertainty • confrontation • alienation • isolation • loneliness • self-absorption • self-pity • incongruence • being unanchored to life • betrayal • powerlessness • grief and loss • insecurity • disenfranchisement • extraordinariness	Becoming ordinary we may experience: • new beginnings • transformation • growth • progress • continuity • confidence • realignment • reconstructing • revising • revaluing • reconnecting • reclaiming • refining • resilience • reconciling • returning to ordinariness • relocation • renewal • healing • wholeness • mastery

before the transition process can begin. Once this acknowledegment occurs one can begin to make sense of what is happening and reorganize a new way to live, respond and be in the world. The process of surfacing awareness involves noticing what has changed and how things are different. Through reflection and introspection people grow stronger and flourish in the brighter opportunities that change has brought into their lives. They locate new ways of living and being in the world that provide the much sought-after sense of meaning, purpose, orientation and inner peace that humans desire. When people begin to see themselves in a new light they may acquaint themselves differently with the person they were before the disruption. People let go of illusions of normality and set about regaining and reclaiming life. A sense of continuity is experienced and ordinariness pervades (box 11.1).

The action process to facilitate transition

Transition entails developing an understanding of disruption in the context of the way life was and becoming ordinary. It is the process that people go through to incorporate the change or disruption into their lives. Transition involves a complex interplay of adaptive activities to manage situational alterations as well as a deeper psychological and spiritual incorporation of changes that aid reorientation of the sense of identity.

Readiness to transition is a complex process of learning, awareness and a reconstruction of self-identity in a way that enables a sense of control and purpose in life. The process of adjustment to the disruption can be a convoluted process interspersed with periods of grief for the perceived loss of the familiar. Shifting perceptions and priorities, altered philosophy and increased self-awareness appear to lead the individual towards a position of reclaiming a sense of control and value as a human being.

The 'look, think, act' process assists people to work out what is going on in their lives, facilitate sense making and reduce ambiguity in their lives. It is a process that facilitates action and provides step by step guidance towards continuity. 'Look, think, act' generally focuses on creating awareness, promoting reflection, and helping to name emotions in order to inform people's thinking process so they choose self-caring responses. The intent of the health worker is to work with people experiencing disruption, to bolster strengths and coping strategies by gently challenging thinking and opening the individual to new possibilities. In our experience, simply creating awareness with disrupted people that they are in a process of learning new ways to becoming ordinary can be enlightening. Guiding people through the 'look, think and act' processes can bring awareness of their uniqueness, strengths and life priorities and provide a guiding framework for people to restructure their goals and take action on those aspects of their lives that are important following the disruption.

In the section to follow we provide some 'look, think and act' prompts that facilitate people to move on. Implicit in this is our search for strengths.

Looking

During this phase the person builds a picture based on information available about what the issue is. From here the person locates the areas to work on to move forwards. The individual is encouraged to take some time to:

- *Describe:*
  What is going on? The circumstances.
  What's happening inside? His/her responses.
- *Gather information to build a picture:*
  Who (the people involved).
  Where (the place).
  When (the time of the situation).
- *Record the information from his/her experiences:*
  Try to get other people's views.
- *Describe the context of what is happening:*
  What thoughts are going on in his/her head?
  How long is he/she mulling over an event afterwards?

Thinking

The individual aims to clarify meaning and increase his/her understanding of the why, when, what, where, how . . . of his/her experiences. Describe the issues and think about what he/she needs to do with/about them. The person may be asked questions like:

- What's the main issue?
- Why is this happening?
- What was the trigger or cause (e.g. attitudes, beliefs, past experiences)?
- What are the consequences?
- How is he/she behaving (e.g. are responses grounded in his/her past)?
- Which area/s can he/she move forward with?
- How might moving forward look?
- When should he/she begin, what order?
- How should he/she do it?
- What are his/her strengths?

Actioning

Thinking about change does not effect change. People can spend a lot of time thinking about what they wish things were like and never take a step towards making change happen. Actioning requires people to become involved with their current situation and choose actions that take them towards their chosen goals. Often there is little choice about the need to change, and one can only choose how to change. A good place to start is to think about what could/should be done differently to get the outcome desired. Then the person could begin to action the smallest and most easily managed act that would have the most benefit to his/her happiness and well being.

People are encouraged to set themselves personal goals and tasks and work out how they will take action on the changes they wish to make. In this step people make an action plan and start the action steps that will help them achieve their plan (Box 11.2).

- What area/s does he/she want to act on first?
- What is most important to him/her right now?
- What is the most achievable thing he/she can act on right now?
- What's the likely outcome of the action?
- What will help him/her to achieve the goal?
- Which people can help?
- Where will the individual find support if needed?

Box 11.2 The changing sense of self in transition: facilitating sense making using the 'look, think and act' process. The issues to explore in the transitional phases.

Look

What's going on? What's happening?

You build a picture based on information available to you about the issues you are dealing with. From here you locate the areas you want/need to work on to move forward.

Describe:
- What is going on?
- What are the circumstances?
- What thoughts are in your head?
- What emotions are being triggered?
- What are your responses?
- Gather information, build a picture:
- Who is involved?
- Where is this change occurring?
- When is it happening?
- Describe the context.
- Try to get other people's views on the situation
- How much are you mulling over the event/experience afterwards?

Think

How am I feeling about it?

Try to get a better understanding and meaning of the issue so that you can work out what you need/want to do about it.

- What is the main issue?
- Why is this happening?
- What do you think is the trigger or cause? (e.g. attitudes, beliefs, past experiences)
- What are the consequences?
- How are you behaving (e.g. are your responses appropriate? Are they reactions that are grounded in the past?)
- In which area/s can you move forward?
- How might this moving forward look?
- When and how should you begin?
- Who can help you?
- Is such a plan possible, given the changes that have occurred?
- What are your strengths? (think about past experiences)
- What might the anticipated consequences and outcomes be?

Focus on your strengths and what is possible in the situation.

Act

What do I want/need to do right now? Who can help? Where? When? How?

Adversity provides little choice about the need to change; you can only choose how you will change. Thinking about change does not effect change. Doing nothing is a choice! Set your personal action goals and then plan how you will make them happen. Become involved with your situation and choose the actions that will take you towards your chosen goals.

- Focus on the opportunities change can bring
- Draw on your past strengths
- Have support people who can reinforce your new patterns of living
- Take specific steps towards your desired outcome
- Do what is most important now
- Start with the smallest thing that is likely to have the most positive impact on your well being with the least work.
- Now take action.

Summary

Participatory action research aims to integrate theory and practice by working *with* people. Furthermore, there has been the need for participatory action research to be focused on developing practical outcomes. This approach is in conflict with most other research approaches, which emphasize the development of theory and are less concerned with practical outcomes or change.

Using participatory action research principles has enabled us to work with people on an equitable basis in the process of knowledge creation. The inclusion of multiple views and perspectives has led us to produce theory that has practical application. Our approach is primarily concerned with practical outcomes or change, and theory development is a bonus, achieved through our exposure to the lives of those with whom we research.

Appendix 1: An example of extracting significant statements from an interview with Albert Baker (Koch, unpublished PhD, 1993)

We felt that it was important to show the way in which significant statements were extracted, and we give below an example of this process, using data generated with Albert Baker, who had been admitted to the care of the elderly ward in an acute care hospital in the United Kingdom. He was interviewed, the recording was transcribed, and analysis begun. At this stage we are extracting significant statements about his experiences in wards designated for older people. He said:

(1) **The typical day was a bore**. I used to wake up about half past 6, 7 o'clock. I was able to walk. I went and had a shave and a wash, you know. But the rest were dished out with bowls and half an inch of water. And from that about 8 o'clock, quarter past 8, the breakfast came. That is all you want, you know, plates of cornflakes or porridge, and a bread roll . . . That takes you to about 9 o'clock. I read, if the doctor wasn't coming, I read until morning tea. Usually that comes at 12 o'clock. So it's one thing on top of another you know. Breakfast is about 8, and the next drink is at 10.30 but it is often 11.30. It is close to lunch.

(2) **I didn't eat** many of the lunches. They tend to be stone cold in the ward. The trolley has to come to the top floor, and then there is the plugging in that they forgot to do many a time. I never saw a menu. My daughter brought in sandwiches for me. Nothing happened until 3 o'clock, the afternoon tea came round. All I did was read and listen to the radio. And at 5 o'clock it was tea time. Once again it was a hot meal, it was a cooked meal, stone cold, as usual. The soups were good though, with my sandwiches. My daughter brought in bananas, oranges and apples.

(3) The **noise at night** was terrific... You know, the shouting. Nobody tried to subdue it you know. I didn't get one night good rest. If I got to sleep at 11 p.m., I would be awakened at 2 or 3 o'clock every night... by the noise... patients shouting out!

(4) **No information. None**: Then they took bone marrow and that nearly killed me. A bone marrow extraction. That was a terrible experience... That young doctor.... I don't know, I don't think she knew what she was doing. I could feel it going in, you know, and she was rolling it about, pump it out, and that was the muddle, and then she pushed it back again and got the blood out, a blood sample, and well I've never witnessed pain like it in my life. No I wasn't prepared for it, I thought it would be like an 'epidermic' or something, but it was a needle about this long. Right to the base of my spine you know. **No information. None.** Just that they were going to take this test, this marrow. I had just come from the ablutions, I had washed and shaved you know. She was waiting, Dr X, at the bed. The doctors... Yes, they don't speak to you, you know.

(5) **I just felt trapped**: I still had flu you know, when I came out. I tried to cover it up so, so they wouldn't keep me in. That's how I felt, after 6 weeks. **I just felt trapped**. Bored to death. And as I say, I was getting no treatment so I might as well have been at home, you know. I wouldn't mind, but really nothing has been done for me, you know. I spent 6 weeks in there but nothing been done. My hands are just the same as when I went in. And my legs are worse.

(6) **I was inside**: They gave me these things when I went home (drugs/vitamins), and I should have been on those while **I was inside**. The day I came out they went down to the pharmacy, a big fancy bag, multivitamins, senna tablets, folic acid, all in nice bottles, you know. I had none of that while I was in there.

(7) **Not a good experience**: You see when I came out of there I dismissed that bloody place from my mind. I dismissed the whole place you know. **Not a good experience**, I don't suppose hospitals are, are they?

(8) **She didn't talk down to me**: To me the best nurses, and there were only two, were A and B. They made an impression on me. If you complained about something, they would do something about it, you know. Not just palm you off, or say I'll see to you later. They actually did it. A did quite a few things for me. For instance, going home, I was asked to see the physio people, before they would let me out. To see if I was capable of walking. And

you know, she arranged things like that. And B, the nurse on night duty, would wake me up in the morning with a cup of tea. She made you feel special. And **she didn't talk down to you** or talk at you. A lot of them talk down to you there, don't they? I don't know whether you have noticed it. I mean that C and that D, they talk down to you, you know. They say: I'm Sister, and I'm Staff... you know. It used to be like that in hospitals, but not these days you know. Things have eased up, haven't they? Nurses should be caring, I think they should be caring, having a bit of sympathy with you, you know, I mean most of those nurses had no sympathy... Show a bit of respect for you, they were cheeky buggers, some of them. Trying to talk down to you, I wouldn't have it though. We are all individuals.

(9) **Just a job**: Casual, the way they go about things you know. A job, it is **just a job**, they come there for the money. Yes there are exceptions but most of it was just top show. They just had to be nice to the patient because there were witnesses there, on a lot of occasions.

(10) **We'll see to you in a few minutes**: Another thing was... taking people to the toilets, people hanging about, asking the nurse could they go to the toilet. 'Oh yes **we'll see to you in a few minutes**' you know, probably it would be 10 minutes or a quarter of an hour after. And it was a lot of trouble to them, you know. It happened often.

(11) **I had one bath in 6 weeks**: The worst of the lot was... that **I had one bath** whilst I was **in** there **6 weeks**. Because... I got bathed the first week, and then the health and safety people from the hospital decided to take all the handles off the hot taps. Not only that, they got lost! So... and they couldn't get any from the works department, so there was no bath for anybody. I had to wash down in the toilets, you know.

About what really mattered to him he said:

(12) **Patients left without food**: The way the **patients** that couldn't feed themselves, quite often got **left without food**, the food was there, but nobody to give it to them, you know. It's true, I watched, what was his name, the chap opposite me... his wife used to come in everyday... Remember him? I've seen him miss his meal dozens of times. And his drink, or you know, his tea, what ever it was he had... because nobody would give it to him. Yes it does concern me really.

(13)   **Death buggy**: I mean seeing . . . there were enough deaths in there, in my short time, there were 13 in there you know. And you know, I saw one chap starve to death . . . I think honestly . . . he came in on the Sunday afternoon and by the Friday he was dead, and nobody had fed him in that time. I watched purposely. He hadn't been fed; he still should have been fed. He died on the Friday. What I didn't like was that **death buggy** coming down for the bodies. Did you ever witness that? It was a big . . . well it was like a steel casket, by the sound of it. And it had iron wheels on it and you pull all the curtains over for everybody, and then they wheel this thing in, you know. Depressing thought.

(14)   **Nobody ever came to see them**: People there they got no relations, you know, I don't know what it was like, it must have been terrible. **Nobody ever came to see them**, you know. It must have been terrible, that. I could think of one or two patients for whom it must have been terrible, but they died. Trying to think of the name of that chap, opposite me, that big chap and he kept sliding out of his chair, do you remember him? He couldn't speak; he'd had a stroke or something. Yes he died, yes. He was one of the deaths . . . Just looking at him you would have thought nothing was wrong with him, you know. He wasn't looked after. He was one that didn't get his drink. It makes me feel . . . you know . . . I was annoyed.

(15)   **It is for old people of course**: People in the ward, no conversation, you know, nothing to say, none of them. **It is for old people of course**, I couldn't talk to anybody with any sense, you know. I can't think of one person that you could talk to. You couldn't get into conversation, they were that ill, most of them.

This is an example of the process of selecting significant statements (in bold) and the evidence to support their utterances. Box A.1 (see below) summarizes the significant statements, grouped according to the questions asked.

A story line can be built from these significant statements and then is it Albert's turn to read and co-construct his story.

Box A.1 Summary of significant statements: Albert Baker.

Significant statements from the response to the question 'what is it like?':

  (1)   The typical day was a bore.
  (2)   I didn't eat.
  (3)   Noise at night.
  (4)   No information. None.
  (5)   I just felt trapped.
  (6)   I was inside.
  (7)   Not a good experience.
  (8)   She didn't talk down to me.
  (9)   Just a job.
 (10)   We'll see to you in a few minutes.
 (11)   I had one bath in 6 weeks.

What matters?

 (12)   Patients left without food.
 (13)   Death buggy.
 (14)   Nobody ever came to see them.
 (15)   It is for old people of course.

Appendix 2: The 'common survivor's story'

An example of a common story line co-constructed with participants of a participatory action research group with Dr Anne van Loon and women who have been sexually abused as children

We were told throughout our lives that we were 'useless', 'good for nothing' and 'deserving of everything we got'. This was reinforced by 'betrayal' from our family and 'manipulation' from the perpetrator/s who 'dominated' us from their position of power and trust, making us feel 'powerless', 'worthless', 'ashamed', 'guilty' and 'to blame somehow'. We were 'used' and treated as 'objects' or 'meat'. When other children were developing 'the building blocks for a strong identity' and understanding that they were unique and worthwhile, able and OK, we were 'stuck' in a world that taught us 'we would never amount to anything'. But worse, we still carry the burden of 'shame' and 'guilt', 'confusion' and 'sadness', which continually diminishes our 'self-worth' and 'shatters our identity'.

We spent our childhood maintaining a shroud of 'silence and secrecy' around our perverse experiences of child sexual abuse. We coped by 'suppressing memories', 'learning to forget', 'disengaging', dis-associating', 'isolating ourselves emotionally and relationally', 'trying to please everyone', 'trying to adapt' and accommodate our 'weird' situation because there was 'no escape anyway'. This allowed us to survive our childhood. But as we became teenagers we came 'unstuck'. We knew we 'didn't fit in'. So we 'numbed our rotten feelings' by taking alcohol, drugs and/or gambling.

For some of us self-harm and re-victimization continued. Weak 'boundaries' made us 'an easy target' for 'predatory people', increasing our 'hopelessness and sadness'. We no longer trusted easily because 'everyone seemed to want something from us' so we chose to become 'disconnected' to protect ourselves from further 'hurt'. We had 'few dreams or hopes for the future', using addictions to 'escape', 'cope' and even 'survive'. We recognize these were 'toxic life patterns'.

When we encounter health professionals we want them to help us with 'sensitivity', 'understanding', 'respect' and 'support' so we can 'heal and grow' towards the future that was 'taken from us during childhood'. We were 'victims', but we have become 'survivors', and with help we are daring to hope and believe we can eventually 'thrive'.

References

Ancoli-Israel, S., Moore, P.J. & Jones, V. (2001) The relationship between fatigue and sleep in cancer patients: a review. *European Journal of Cancer Care*, **10** (4), 245–255.

Atkinson, P. (1995) *Medical Talk and Medical Work*. Sage Publications, London.

Austin, W., Bergum, V. & Dossetor, J. (2003) Relational ethics: an action ethic as a foundation for health care. In: V. Tschudin (Ed) *Approaches to Ethics*. Butterworth Heinemann, Toronto.

Banister, E. (1999) Evolving reflexivity: negotiating meaning of women's midlife experience. *Qualitative Inquiry*, **5** (1), 3–23.

Barnard, D., Towers, A., Boston, P. & Lambrinidou, Y. (2000) *Crossing Over: Narratives of Palliative Care*. Oxford University Press, New York.

Bartlett, M.C., Brauner, D.J., Coats, B.C., England, S.E., Gaibel, I., Ganzer, C., Gorman, J., Graham, M.E., Marder, R., Miller, B., O'Shea, B. & Poirier, S. (1993) Moral reasoning and Alzheimer's care: exploring complex weavings through narrative. *Journal of Aging Studies*, **7** (4), 409–421.

Beauchamp, T. & Childress, J. (2001) *Principles of Biomedical Ethics* (5th edn). Oxford University Press, New York.

Becker, G. (1997) *Disrupted Lives: How People Create Meaning on a Chaotic World*. University of California Press, Berkeley.

Belenky, M., Clincy, B., Goldberger, N. & Tarule, J. (1986) *Women's Ways of Knowing*. Basic Books, New York.

Berube, M. (1996) *Life as We Know It: a Father, a Family, and an Exceptional Child*. Random House, New York.

Bhavnani, K. (1988) What's power got to do with it? Empowerment and social research. *Text*, **8**, 41–50.

Bowes, A. (1996) Evaluating an empowering research strategy: reflections on action-research with south Asian women. *Sociological Research Online* 1 (1). http://www.socre sonline.org.uk/socresonline/1/1/1.html

Bray, J., Lee, J., Smith, L. & Yorks, L. (2000) *Collaborative Inquiry in Practice*. Sage Publications, London.

Bridges, W. (1980) *Transitions: Making Sense of Life's Changes*. Addison-Wesley, New York.

Bridges, W. (2004) *Transitions: Making Sense of Life's Changes* (2nd edn). Da Capo Press, Cambridge, Massachusetts.

Brody, H. (2003) *Stories of Sickness*. Oxford University Press, New York.

Bruner, J. (2002) *Making Stories: Law, Literature, Life*. First Harvard University Press, Harvard.

Burdekin, B. (1993) *Human Rights and Mental Illness: Report to the National Inquiry into the Human Rights of People with Mental Illness*. Human Rights and Equal Opportunity Commission, Canberra, Australia.

Bury, M. (1982) Chronic illness as biographical disruption. *Sociology of Health and Illness*, **4**, 167–182.

Bury, M. (1991) The sociology of chronic illness: a review of research and prospects. *Sociology of Health and Illness*, **13** (4), 451–468.

Cancian, F. (1992) Participatory research. In: E.F. Borgatta and M. Borgatta (Eds). *Encyclopedia of Sociology* (pp. 1427–1432). Macmillan, New York.

Cancian, F. & Armstead, C. (1990) *Participatory Research: An Introduction*. Department of Sociology, University of California, Irvine, California.

Cantanzaro, M. (1990) Transitions in midlife adults with long-term illness. *Holistic Nurse Practitioner* **4** (3), 65–73.

Chambers, T. (1999) *The Fiction of Bioethics*. Routledge, New York.

Charmaz, K. (1983) Loss of self: a fundamental form of suffering in the chronically ill. *Sociology of Health and Illness*, **5**, 168–195.

Charon, R. & Montello, M. (2002) Introduction. In: R. Charon & M. Montello (Eds) *Stories Matter: The Role of Narrative in Medical Ethics*. Routledge, New York.

Chick, N. & Meleis, A.I. (1986) Transitions: a nursing concern. In: P.L. Chinn (Ed) *Nursing Research Methodology: Issues and Implementation* (pp. 237–257). Aspen, Rockville, Maryland.

Chinn, P. (2003) Feminist approaches. In: J. Clare & H. Hamilton (Eds) *Writing Research* (pp. 61–85). Churchill Livingstone, London.

Chinn, P. & Kramer, M. (1999) *Theory and Nursing, Integrated Knowledge Development* (5th edn). Mosby, Elsevier, Sydney.

Coffey, M. (1998) Schizophrenia: a review of current research and thinking. *Journal of Clinical Nursing*, **7** (6), 489–498.

Coles, R. (1989) *The Call of Stories: Teaching and the Moral Imagination*. Houghton Mifflin, Boston.

Corbin, J. & Strauss, A. (1987) Accompaniments of chronic illness: change in the body, self, biography and biographical time. *Research in the Sociology of Health Care*, **6**, 249–281.

Couser, G.T. (1997) *Recovering Bodies: Illness, Disability and Life Writing*. The University of Wisconsin Press, Madison, Wisconsin.

Cowles, K. (1988) Issues in qualitative research on sensitive topics. *Western Journal of Nursing Research*, **10**, 163–179.

Crossley, M.L. (2000) *Introducing Narrative Psychology: Self, Trauma and the Construction of Meaning*. Open University Press, Buckingham.

Cruikshank, J., Sidney, A., Smith, K. & Ned, A. (1992) *Life Lived Like a Story*. University of Nebraska Press, Lincoln.

De Raeve, L. (1994) Ethical issues in palliative care research. *Palliative Medicine*, **8**, 298–305.

DeRenzo, E. (1998) Power differentials, context, relationship, and emotions: feminist ethics. Considerations and human subjects research. *Journal of Womens Health*, **7** (8), 971–977.

Dewey, J. (1933) *How we Think: a Restatement of the Relation of Reflective Thinking to the Educative Process*. Heath, Boston.

Diabetes Australia (1998) *National Diabetes Strategy*.
http://www.diabetes.net.au/national_diabetes_programs/australia.asp

Dick, B. (2004) Action research literature themes and trends. *Action Research*, **2** (4), 425–444.

Duffy, M. (1985) A critique of research: a feminist perspective. *Health Care for Women International*, **6**, 341–352.

Eakin, P.J. (1999) *How Our Lives Become Stories: Making Selves*. Cornell University Press, Ithica.

Eastwood, S., Kralik, D. & Koch, T. (2002) Compromising and containing: self-management strategies used by men and women who live with multiple sclerosis and urinary incontinence. *The Australian Journal of Holistic Nursing*, **9** (1), 33–43.

Erlandson, D., Harris, E., Skipper, B. & Allen, S. (1993) *Doing Naturalistic Inquiry: a Guide to Methods*. Sage Publications, Thousand Oaks, California.

Estroff, S. (1995) Whose story is it anyway? Authority, voice and responsibility in chronic illness. In: S. Toombs, D. Barnard & R. Carson (Eds) *Chronic Illness: From Experience to Policy* (pp. 77–102). Indiana University Press, Bloomington.

Fals Borda, O. (2001) Participatory (action) research in social theory: origin and challenges. In: P. Reason & H. Bradbury (Eds) *Handbook of Action Research* (pp. 27–37). Sage Publications, Thousand Oaks, California.

Faulkner, A. (1980) Nursing as a research-based profession. *Nursing Focus*, August, 477.

Field, D. (1989) *Nursing the Dying*. Travistock/Routledge, London.

Finch, J. (1984) It's great to have someone to talk to: the ethics and politics of interviewing women. In: C. Bell & H. Roberts (Eds) *Social Researching: Politics, Problems, Practice* (pp. 70–87). Routledge and Kegan Paul, London.

FitzGerald, M. (1997) Nursing and researching. *International Journal of Nursing Practice* **3** (1), 53–56.

Ford, J. & Reutter, L. (1990) Ethical dilemmas associated with small samples. *Journal of Advanced Nursing*, **15**, 187–191.

Frank, A.W. (1993) The rhetoric of self-change: illness experience as narrative. *Sociological Quarterly*, **34** (1), 39–52.

Frank, A.W. (1995) *The Wounded Storyteller*. University of Chicago Press, Chicago.

Freire, P. (1970) *Pedagogy of the Oppressed*. Translated by Myra Bergman Ramos for Penguin Books in 1996. Penguin Books, Harmondsworth.

Friedlander, F. (1982) Alternative modes of inquiry. *Small Group Behaviour*, **13** (400), 428–440.

Gadamer, H.-G. (1976) *Philosophical Hermeneutics*. University of California Press, Berkeley.

Gadamer, H.-G. (1989) *Truth and Method*. The Crossroad Publishing Corporation, New York.

Garro, L.C. & Mattingly, C. (2000) Narrative as construct and construction. In: C. Mattingly & L.C. Garro (Eds) *Narrative and the Cultural Construction of Illness and Healing*. University of California Press, Berkeley, California.

Gaventa, J. & Cornwall, A. (2001) Theory and practice: the mediating discourse. In: P. Reason & H. Bradbury (Eds) *Handbook of Action Research* (pp. 70–80). Sage, Thousand Oaks, California.

Gergen, K. (1991) *The Saturated Self: Dilemmas of Identity in Contemporary Life*. Basic Books, New York.

Gergen, K. (1999) *An Invitation to Social Construction*. Sage Publications, Thousand Oaks, California.

Gergen, K. (2003) Action research and orders of democracy. *Action Research*, **1** (1), 39–56.

Gobodo-Madikizela, P. (2004) *A Human Being Died that Night*. Houghton Mifflin, New York.

Gramsci, A. (1971) *Selection from Prison Notebooks*. New York International Publishers, New York.

Green, L.W., George, M.A., Daniel, M., Frankish, C.J., Herbert, C.P., Bowie, W.R. & O'Neill, M. (2003) Appendix C: guidelines for participatory research in health promotion. In: M. Minkler & N. Wallerstein (Eds) *Community-Based Participatory Research for Health*. Jossey-Bass, San Francisco, California.

Guba, E. & Lincoln, Y. (1989) *Fourth Generation Evaluation*. Sage Publications, Thousand Oaks, California.

Gustavsen, B. (2001) Theory and practice: the mediating discourse. In: P. Reason & H. Bradbury (Eds) *Handbook of Action Research* (pp. 17–26). Sage Publications, Thousand Oaks, California.

Hagey, R. (1997) The use and abuse of participatory action research. *Chronic Diseases in Canada*, **18** (1). http:/www.hc-sc.gc.ca/pphb-dgspsp/publicat/cdic-mcc/18-1/a_e.html

Hall, B. (2001) I wish this were a poem of practices of participatory research. In: P. Reason & H. Bradbury (Eds) *Handbook of Action Research* (pp. 171–178). Sage Publications, Thousand Oaks, California.

Henderson, D. (1995) Consciousness raising in participatory research: method and methodology for emancipatory nursing inquiry. *Advances in Nursing Science*, **17** (3), 58–69.

Heron, J. & Reason, P. (2001) The practice of cooperative inquiry: research 'with' rather than 'on' people. In: P. Reason & H. Bradbury (Eds) *Handbook of Action Research*. Sage Publications, Thousands Oaks, California.

Hiebert, J. (1996) Learning circles: a strategy for clinical practicum. *Nurse Educator*, **21** (3), 37–42.

Holloway, I. (1997) *Basic Concepts for Qualitative Research*. Blackwell Science, Oxford.

Holstein, J. & Gubrium, J. (2000) *The Self we Live By: Narrative Identity in a Postmodern World*. Oxford University Press, New York.

Horowitz, M. (1976) *Stress Response Syndromes*. Jason Aronson, New York.

Hudson, S. (1999) Ethics for alternative paradgims: an exploration of options. *Graduate Research Nursing*, October. http://www.graduateresearch.com/hudson.htm

Hutchinson, S., Wilson, M. & Skodol Wilson, H. (1994) Benefits of participating in research interviews. *Image: Journal of Nursing Scholarship*, **26** (2), 161–164.

Israel, B., Schultz, A., Parker, E. & Becker, A. (1998) Review of community-based research: assessing partnership approaches to improve public health. *Annual Review of Public Health*, **19**, 173–202.

Jenkin, P. & Koch, T. (2004) The experience of fatigue and strategies for self-management among community-dwelling persons living with HIV. *Royal District Nursing Service Research Unit*. RDNS Foundation, Glenside, South Australia. http://www.rdns.net.au

Kavanaugh, K. & Ayres, L. (1998) 'Not as bad as it could have been': assessing and mitigating harm during research interviews on sensitive topics. *Research in Nursing and Health*, **21**, 91–97.

Kelly, M. & Field, D. (1996) Medical sociology, chronic illness and the body. *Sociology of Health and Illness*, **18** (2), 241–257.

Kemmis, S. (2001) Exploring the relevance of clinical theory for action research: emancipatory action research in the footsteps of Jurgen Habermas. In: P. Reason & H. Bradbury (Eds) *Handbook of Action Research* (pp. 91–102). Sage Publications, Thousand Oaks, California.

Kemmis, S. & McTaggert, R. (1988) *The Action Research Planner* (3rd edn). Deakin University, Victoria, Australia.

Kemmis, S. & McTaggart, R. (1988) Introduction: the nature of action research. In: S. Kemmis & S. McTaggart (Eds) *The Action Research Planner* (3rd edn) (pp. 5–28). Deakin University, Australia.

Kimberley Aboriginal Medical Services West Australia (1998) *Systematic Review of the Evidence and Primary Care Guidelines on the Management of Non-Insulin Dependent Diabetes in Aboriginal and Torres Strait Islander Populations.* Commonwealth Department of Health and Family Services for the Office for Aboriginal and Torres Strait Islander Health, Canberra.

Kleinman, A. (1988) *The Illness Narratives: Suffering and the Human Condition.* Basic Books, New York.

Kleinman, A., Brodwin, P.E., Good, B.J. & Good, M.-J.D. (1992) Pain as human experience – an introduction. In: M.-J.D. Good, P.E. Brodwin, B.J. Good & A. Kleinman (Eds) *Pain as Human Experience – An Anthropological Perspective.* University of California Press, Berkeley, California.

Koch, T. (1993) *Towards fourth generation evaluation: listening to the voices of older patients. A hermeneutic inquiry.* Unpublished PhD thesis. University of Manchester.

Koch, T. (1994) Establishing rigour in qualitative research: the decision trail. *Journal of Advanced Nursing*, **19**, 976–986.

Koch, T. (1996) Implementation of a hermeneutic inquiry in nursing: philosophy, rigour and representation. *Journal of Advanced Nursing*, **24**, 174–184.

Koch, T. (1998) Story telling: is it really research? *Journal of Advanced Nursing*, **28** (6), 1182–1190.

Koch, T. (2003) Collaborative evaluation research. In: Z. Schneider, D. Elliott, G. LoBiondo-Wood & J. Haber (Eds) *Nursing Research: Methods, Critical Appraisal and Utilisation* (2nd edn) (pp. 233–245). Elsevier (Australia), Sydney.

Koch, T. & Harrington, A. (1998) Reconceptualizing rigour: the case for reflexivity. *Journal of Advanced Nursing*, **28** (4), 882–890.

Koch, T. & Kralik, D. (2002) Development of a collaborative model of care for long term management of incontinence for people living in the community with mental illness. *Royal District Nursing Service Research Unit.* RDNS Foundation, Glenside, South Australia. http://www.rdns.net.au

Koch, T., Kralik, D. & Sonnack, D. (1999) Women living with type 2 diabetes: the intrusion of illness. *Journal of Clinical Nursing*, **8**, 712–722.

Koch, T., Kralik, D. & Taylor, J. (1999) Men living with diabetes: minimising the intrusiveness of the disease. *Journal of Clinical Nursing*, **9**, 247–254.

Koch, T., Kralik, D. & Eastwood, S. (2002) Constructions of sexuality for women living with multiple sclerosis. *Journal of Advanced Nursing*, **39** (2), 137–145.

Koch, T., Jenkin, P. & Kralik, D. (2003) Development of a collaborative asthma management model for older people living in the community. *Royal District Nursing Service Research Unit*. RDNS Foundation, Glenside, South Australia. http://www.rdns.net.au

Koch, T., Jenkin, P. & Kralik, D. (2004) Chronic illness self-management: locating the 'self'. *Journal of Advanced Nursing*, **48** (5), 484–492.

Koch, T., Jenkins, P. & Kralik, D. (2006) Experience of fatigue for adults living with HIV. *Journal of Clinical Nursing*, in press.

KPMG Management Consulting (1997) *National Evaluation of the Aboriginal and Torres Strait Islander Coordinated Care Trials*. KPMG Management Consulting, Adelaide.

Kralik, D. (2000) *The quest for ordinariness: midlife women living through chronic illness*. Unpublished PhD thesis, Flinders University of South Australia, Adelaide.

Kralik, D. (2002) The quest for ordinariness: transition experienced by midlife women living with chronic illness. *Journal of Advanced Nursing*, **39** (2), 146–154.

Kralik, D. (2005) Participatory approach in feminist research. In: I. Holloway (Ed) *Qualitative Research for the Health Professions* (pp. 250–269). Open University Press, Milton Keynes.

Kralik, D., Koch, T. & Wotton, K. (1997) Engagement and detachment: understanding patients experiences with nursing. *Journal of Advanced Nursing*, **26**, 399–407.

Kralik, D., Koch, T. & Brady, B.M. (2000) Pen pals: correspondence as a method for data generation in qualitative research. *Journal of Advanced Nursing*, **31** (4), 909–917.

Kralik, D., Koch, T. & Telford, K. (2001a) Constructions of sexuality for midlife women living with chronic illness. *Journal of Advanced Nursing*, **35** (2), 180–187.

Kralik, D., Koch, T. & Webb, C. (2001b) The domination of chronic illness research by biomedical interests. *Australian Journal of Holistic Nursing*, **8** (2), 4–12.

Kralik, D., Koch, T. & Eastwood, S. (2003) The salience of the body: transition in sexual self-identity for women living with multiple sclerosis. *Journal of Advanced Nursing*, **42** (1), 11–20.

Kralik, D., Koch, T., Price, K. & Howard, N. (2004) Chronic illness self-management: taking action to create order. *Journal of Clinical Nursing*, **13** (2), 259–267.

Kralik, D., Price, K., Warren, J. & Koch, T. (2006) Email group conversations as data for nursing research. *Journal of Advanced Nursing*, **53**(2), 213–20.

Lather, P. (1988) Feminist perspectives on empowering research methodologies. *Women's Studies International Forum*, **56** (3), 257–277.

Lather, P. (1991) *Getting Smart: Feminist Research and Pedagogy Within the Postmodern*. Routledge, New York.

Lawrence, E. (1982) In the abundance of water, the fool is thirsty: sociology and black 'pathology'. In: Centre for Contemporary Cultural Studies (Eds) *The Empire Strikes Back: Race and Racism in 70s Britain*. Hutchinson, London.

Lee, K.A., Lentz, M.J., Taylor, D.L., Mitchell, E.S. & Woods, N.F. (1994) Fatigue as a response to environmental demands in women's lives. *Image – the Journal of Nursing Scholarship*, **26** (2), 149–154.

Levine, M. (1977) Nursing ethics and the ethical nurse. *American Journal of Nursing*, **77** (5), 846.

Loveys, B. (1990) Transitions in chronic illness: the at-risk role. *Holistic Nursing Practice*, **4**, 45–64.

MacLean, D. & Lo, R. (1998) The non-insulin dependent diabetic: success and failure in compliance. *Australian Journal of Advanced Nursing*, **15** (4), 33–42.

Macmurray, J. (1961) *Persons in Relation*. Volume 11 of *The Form of the Personal*. Farber & Farber, London.

Maguire, P. (1987) *Doing Participatory Research: a Feminist Approach*. University of Massachusetts, Amherst, Massachusetts.

Maguire, P. (1996) Proposing a more feminist participatory research: knowing and being embraced openly. In: K. de Koning & M. Martin (Eds) *Participatory Research in Health* (pp. 27–39). Zed Books, London.

Maguire, P. (2001) Uneven ground: feminisms and action research. In: P. Reason & H. Bradbury (Eds) *Handbook of Action Research* (pp. 59–69). Sage, London.

Mann, S. (2002) *Participatory action research to improve diabetes self-management with Aboriginal families*. Unpublished report to National Health and Medical Research Australia. A collaborative project between elders from the Port Lincoln Aboriginal Community, Aboriginal health workers and other staff from the Port Lincoln Aboriginal Health Service (PLAHS), the Research Unit at the Royal District Nursing Service SA Inc (RDNS), the Spencer Gulf Health School (SGRHS) and the Eyre Peninsula Division of General Practice (EPDGP), South Australia.

Mann, S. (2003) *Look, think, act using the principles of participatory action for facilitating community groups learning guide*. Research Unit Report (unpublished). Study title: Look, Think and Act: Indigenous Stories about Living with Diabetes. Resource is available in the RDNS Information Centre. Report is available on the RDNS website: www.rdns.org.au

Mann, C. & Stewart, F. (2000) *Internet Communication and Qualitative Research*. Sage, London.

Marrow, A. (1969) *The Practical Theorist: The Life and Work of Kurt Lewin*. Basic Books, New York.

Mattingly, C. (1998) *Healing Dramas and Clinical Plots*. Cambridge University Press, Cambridge.

Mazza, D., Dennerstein, L., Garamszegi, C. & Dudley, E. (2001) The physical, sexual and emotional violence history of middle-aged women: a community-based prevalence study. *Medical Journal of America*, **175**, 199–201.

McArdle, K.L. & Reason, P. (2006) Action research and organization development. In: T. Cummings (Ed) *Handbook of Organization Development*. Sage Publications, Thousand Oaks, California.

Meleis, A.I. & Trangenstein, P.A. (1994) Facilitating transitions: redefinition of the nursing mission. *Nursing Outlook*, **42** (6), 255–259.

Meleis, A.I., Sawyer, L.M., Im, E.-O., Hilfinger Messias, D.K. & Schumacher, K. (2000) Experiencing transitions: an emerging middle-range theory. *Advances in Nursing Science*, **23** (1), 12–28.

Meyer, J. (2000) Using qualitative methods in health related action research. *British Medical Journal*, **320**, 178–181.

Mies, M. (1983) Toward a methodology of feminist research. In: G. Bowles & R. Duelli-Klein (Eds) *Theories of Women's Studies* (pp. 117–139). Routledge and Kegan Paul, Boston.

Miles, A. (1998) *Integrative Feminisms: Building Global Visions 1960s–1990s.* Routledge, New York.

Minkler, M. & Wallerstein, N. (2003) *Community-Based Participatory Research for Health.* Jossey Bass, San Francisco, California.

Mishler, E. (1986) *Research Interviewing: Context and Narrative.* Harvard University Press, Cambridge, Massachusetts.

Morris, D.B. (1993) *The Culture of Pain.* University of California Press, Berkeley, California.

Munhall, P. (1988) Ethical considerations in qualitative research. *Western Journal of Nursing Research*, **10**, 150–162.

Nelson, H.L. (2001) *Damaged Identities, Narrative Repair.* Cornell University Press, Ithaca.

Nettleton, S. & Watson, J. (1998) The body in everyday life: an introduction. In: S. Nettleton & J. Watson (Eds) *The Body in Everyday Life* (pp. 1–24). Aspen, New York.

Nguyen, A., Roder, D., McCaul, K., Priest, K., Carman, J. & Luke, C. (1996) *South Australian Regional Health Statistics Chartbook: A Working Document.* SAHC, Adelaide.

Northway, R. (2000) The relevance of participatory research in developing nursing research and practice. *Nurse Researcher*, **7** (4), 40–52.

Oakley, A. (1981) Interviewing women: a contradiction in terms. In: H. Roberts (Ed) *Doing Feminist Research.* Routledge, London.

Olsen, V. (1994) Feminisms and models of qualitative research. In: N.K. Denzin & Y.S. Lincoln (Eds) *Handbook of Qualitative Research* (pp. 158–174). Sage, Thousand Oaks, California.

Opie, A. (1992) Qualitative research, appropriation of the 'other' and empowerment. *Feminist Review*, **40**, 52–69.

Parker, Z. (1998) PhD students and the auto/biographies of their learning. In: M. Erben (Ed) *Biography and Education.* Falmer, London.

Pasmore, W. (2001) Action research in the workplace: the socio-technical perspective. In: P. Reason & H. Bradbury (Eds) *Handbook of Action Research* (pp. 38–47). Sage Publications, Thousand Oaks, California.

Paterson, B., Thorne, S. & Russell, S. (2002) Disease-specific influences on meaning and significance in self-care decision-making in chronic illness. *Canadian Journal of Nursing Research*, **34** (3), 61–74.

Price, J. (1996) Snakes in the swamp: ethical issues in qualitative research. In: R. Josselson (Ed) *The Narrative Study of Lives: Volume 4. Ethics and Process* (pp. 207–215). Sage Publications, Thousand Oaks, California.

Quas, J., Goodman, G. & Jones, D. (2003) Predictors of attributions of self-blame and internalizing behavior problems in sexually abused children. *Journal of Child Psychology & Psychiatry & Allied Disciplines*, **44**, 723–736.

Reason, P. (1994) Collaborative inquiry. In: N. Denzin & Y. Lincoln (Eds) *Handbook of Qualitative Research* (pp. 324–339). Sage Publications, Thousand Oaks, California.

Reason, P. (1994) Three approaches to participative inquiry. In: N. Denzin & Y. Lincoln (Eds) *Handbook of Qualitative Research* (pp. 324–339). Sage, Thousand Oaks, California.

Reason, P. (1998) Political, epistemological, ecological and spiritual dimensions of participation. *Studies in Cultures, Organizations and Societies*, **4**, 147–167.

Reason, P. (2001) The practice of co-operative inquiry: research with rather than on people (with John Heron). In: P. Reason & H. Bradbury (Eds) *Handbook of Action Research: Participative Inquiry and Practice* (pp. 179–188). Sage, London.

Reason, P. & Bradbury, H. (2001) *Handbook of Action Research: Participatory Inquiry and Practice*. Sage Publications, London.

Redman, B. (2004) *Patient Self-Management of Chronic Disease*. Jones and Bartlett, London.

Reinharz, S. (1992) *Feminist Methods in Social Research*. Oxford University Press, Oxford.

Ribbens, J. (1989) Interviewing women: an unnatural situation. *Women's Studies International Forum*, **112**, 579–592.

Robinson, I. (1995) Personal narratives, social careers and medical courses: analysing life trajectories in autobiographies of people with multiple sclerosis. *Social Science Medicine*, **30** (11), 1173–1186.

Saldana, J. (2003) *Longitudinal Qualitative Research: Analyzing Change Through Time*. AltaMira Press, Oxford.

Schön, D.A. (1983) *How Professionals Think in Action*. Basic Books, New York.

Schön, D. (1991) *The Reflective Practitioner: How Professionals Think in Action*. Ashgate Publishing, Avebury.

Schumacher, K.L. & Meleis, A.I. (1994) Transistions: a central concept in nursing. *IMAGE: Journal of Nursing Scholarship*, **26** (2), 119–127.

Sclater, S.D. (1998) Stories as transitional phenomena. *Auto/Biography*, **6** (1 and 2), 85–92.

Seibold, C., Richards, L. & Simon, D. (1994) Feminist method and qualitative research about midlife. *Journal of Advanced Nursing*, **19**, 394–402.

Selder, F. (1989) Life transition theory: the resolution of uncertainty. *Nursing & Health Care*, **10** (8), 437–451.

Seng, J. (1998) Praxis as a conceptual framework for participatory research in nursing. *Advances in Nursing Science*, **20** (4), 37–48.

Seymour, J. & Ingelton, C. (1999) Ethical issues in qualitative research at the end of life. *International Journal of Palliative Nursing*, **5** (2), 65–73.

Smith, L. (1992) Ethical issues in interviewing. *Journal of Advanced Nursing*, **17**, 98–103.

Speedy, S. (1991) The contribution of feminist research. In: G. Gray & R. Pratt (Eds) *Towards a Discipline of Nursing*. Churchill Livingstone, Melbourne.

Stanley, L. & Wise, S. (1983) *Breaking Out Again: Feminist Ontology and Epistemology*. Routledge, London.

Street, A. (1995) *Establishing a Participatory Action Group, Nursing Replay: Research Nursing Culture Together, Volume 1*. Churchill Livingstone, Melbourne.

Stringer, E. (1996) *Action Research: a Handbook for Practitioners*. Sage Publications, Thousand Oaks, California.

Stringer, E. (1999) *Action Research: a Handbook for Practitioners* (2nd edn). Sage Publications, Thousand Oaks, California.

Stringer, E. & Genat, W. (2004) *Action Research in Health*. Pearson Education, Upper Saddle River, New Jersey.

Tschudin, V. (2003) Narrative ethics. In: V. Tschudin (Ed) *Approaches to Ethics*. Butterworth Heinemann, Toronto.

Tuckman, B. (1965) Developmental sequence in small groups. *Psychological Bulletin*, **63** (6), 384–399.

Van Manen, M. (1996) From meaning to method. *Qualitative Health Research*, **7** (3), 345–369.

Wadsworth, Y. (1998) *What is participatory action research?* http://www.scu.edu.au/schools/gcm/ar/ari/p-ywadsworth98.html

Waitzkin, H. (1991) *The Politics of Medical Encounters: How Patients and Doctors Deal with Social Problems*. Yale University Press, New Haven.

Wass, A. (2001) *Promoting Health: the Primary Health Care Approach* (2nd edn). Harcourt, Sydney (now Elsevier Publishing).

Webb, C. (1993) Feminist research: definitions, methodology, methods and evaluation. *Journal of Advanced Nursing*, **18**, 416–423.

Weedon, C. (1987) *Feminist Practice and Poststructuralist Theory*. Basil Blackwell, New York.

Winter, R. (1998) Finding voice, thinking with others: a conception of action research. *Educational Action Research*, **6** (1), 53–68.

Yoshida, K. (1994) Institutional impact on self concept among persons with spinal cord injury. *International Journal of Rehabilitation Research*, **17** (2), 95–107.

Index